CW00403020

KETO
MEAL PREP

*Lose Weight and Stay in Shape with
the Right Nutrition*

MAX LOREN

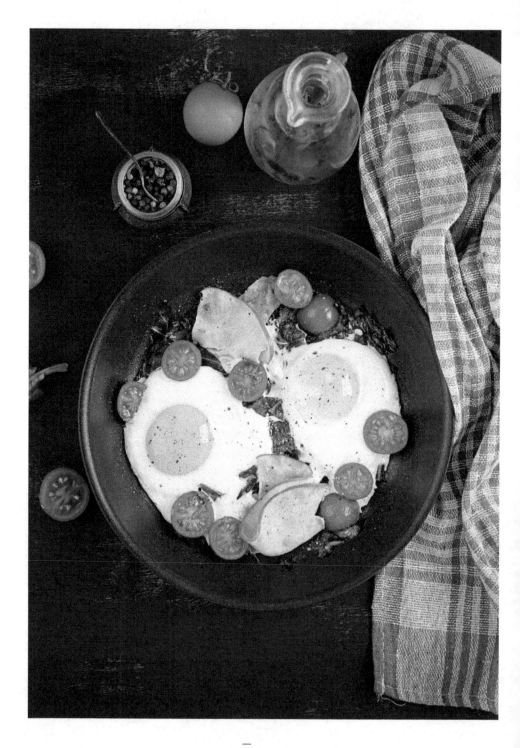

©**Copyright 2021 - All rights reserved.**
The content contained within this book may not be reproduced, duplicated or transmitted without direct written permission from the author or the publisher.

Under no circumstances will any blame or legal responsibility be held against the publisher, or author, for any damages, reparation, or monetary loss due to the information contained within this book. Either directly or indirectly.

Legal Notice:

This book is copyright protected. This book is only for personal use. You cannot amend, distribute, sell, use, quote or paraphrase any part, or the content within this book, without the consent of the author or publisher.

Disclaimer Notice:

Please note the information contained within this document is for educational and entertainment purposes only. All effort has been executed to present accurate, up to date, and reliable, complete information. No warranties of any kind are declared or implied. Readers acknowledge that the author is not engaging in the rendering of legal, financial, medical or professional advice. The content within this book has been derived from various sources. Please consult a licensed professional before attempting any techniques outlined in this book.

By reading this document, the reader agrees that under no circumstances is the author responsible for any losses, direct or indirect, which are incurred as a result of the use of information contained within this document, including, but not limited to, errors, omissions, or inaccuracies.

Table of Contents

Sommario

—

Introduction

The ketogenic diet, or keto diet, is a low-carbohydrate, high-fat diet that provides many health benefits.Many studies have shown that this type of diet can help you reduce and improve your health.Ketogenic diets may even have benefits against diabetes, cancer, epilepsy, and Alzheimer's disease.

What is a ketogenic diet?

The ketogenic diet is a low carbohydrate, high-fat diet that has many similarities to the Atkins and low carb diets.It involves drastically reducing carbohydrate intake and replacing carbohydrates with fat. This drastic reduction in carbs puts your body into a metabolic state called ketosis.When this occurs, your body is incredibly efficient at burning fat for energy. It also converts fat into ketones within the liver, which can form the energy for the brain.Ketogenic diets can cause major reductions in blood glucose and insulin levels. This, along with the increase in ketones, has health benefits.

Different types of ketogenic diets

There are several versions of the ketogenic diet, including:

The standard ketogenic diet (SKD): This is often a low carb, moderate protein, and high-fat diet. It typically contains 70% fat, 20% protein, and only 10% carbs (9Trusted Source).

The cyclical ketogenic diet (CKD): This diet involves periods of upper carb refeeds, like 5 ketogenic days followed by 2 high carb days.

The targeted ketogenic diet (TKD): This diet allows you to feature carbs around workouts.

High protein ketogenic diet: this is often almost like a typical ketogenic diet, but includes more protein. The ratio is usually 60% fat, 35% protein, and 5% carbs.

However, only the quality and high protein ketogenic diets are studied extensively. Cyclical or targeted ketogenic diets are more advanced methods and are primarily employed by bodybuilders or athletes.

What is ketosis?

Ketosis may be a metabolic state during which your body uses fat for fuel rather than carbs.

It occurs once you significantly reduce your consumption of carbohydrates, limiting your body's supply of glucose (sugar), which is that the main source of energy for the cells.

Following a ketogenic diet is that the best thanks to entering ketosis. Generally, this involves limiting carb consumption to around 20 to 50 grams per day and filling abreast of fats, like meat, fish, eggs, nuts, and healthy oils

It's also important to moderate your protein consumption, this is often because protein can be converted into glucose if consumed in high amounts, which can slow your transition into ketosis

Practicing intermittent fasting could also assist you to enter ketosis faster. There are many various sorts of intermittent fasting, but the foremost common method involves limiting food intake to around 8 hours per day and fasting for the remaining 16 hours

Blood, urine, and breath tests are available, which may help determine whether you've entered ketosis by measuring the number of ketones produced by your body.

Certain symptoms can also indicate that you've entered ketosis, including increased thirst, dry mouth, frequent urination, and decreased hunger or appetite

Ketogenic diets can help you lose weight

A ketogenic diet is also an effective solution for losing weight and decreasing risk factors for disease.

Research has shown that the ketogenic diet can be very effective for weight loss as a low-fat diet.

What's more, the diet is so rich that you can lose weight without needing to count calories or track your food intake.

An analysis of 13 studies revealed that following a low-carb ketogenic diet was slightly superior for long-term weight loss compared to a low-fat diet.

It also led to a reduction in diastolic blood pressure and triglyceride levels.

Other health benefits of keto

- The ketogenic diet originated as a method of treating neurological diseases such as epilepsy.
- Studies have now shown that this diet may have benefits for a wide variety of different health conditions:

- Heart disease. The ketogenic diet can help improve risk factors such as body fat, HDL (good) cholesterol levels, blood pressure, and blood sugar.

- Cancer. Diet is currently being explored as an adjunct treatment for cancer because it may help slow tumor growth.

- Alzheimer's disease. The keto diet may help reduce the symptoms of Alzheimer's disease and slow its progression.

- Epilepsy. Research has shown that the ketogenic diet can cause significant reductions in seizures in epileptic children.

- Parkinson's disease. Although more research is needed, one study found that the diet helped improve symptoms of Parkinson's disease.

- Polycystic ovary syndrome. The ketogenic diet may help reduce insulin levels, which may play a key role in polycystic ovary syndrome.

- Brain injury. Some research suggests that the diet may improve the outcomes of traumatic brain injuries.

However, keep in mind that research in many of these areas is far from conclusive.

Foods to avoid

Any food high in carbohydrates should be reduced.

Here is a list of foods that should be reduced or eliminated on a ketogenic diet:

sugary foods: soda, juice, smoothies, cake, ice cream, candy, etc.

grains or starches: wheat products, rice, pasta, cereals, etc.

fruits: all fruits, except small portions of berries such as strawberries

beans or legumes: peas, beans, lentils, chickpeas, etc.

root and tuber vegetables: potatoes, sweet potatoes, carrots, parsnips, etc.

low-fat or diet products: low-fat mayonnaise, salad dressings, and condiments

some condiments or sauces: barbecue sauce, honey mustard, teriyaki sauce, ketchup, etc.

unhealthy fats: processed vegetable oils, mayonnaise, etc.

alcohol: beer, wine, liquor, mixed drinks

sugar-free diet foods: sugar-free candy, syrups, puddings, sweeteners, desserts, etc.

Foods to eat

You should focus most of your meals on these foods:

meat: red meat, steak, ham, sausage, bacon, chicken, and turkey

fatty fish: salmon, trout, tuna, and mackerel

eggs: whole pastured eggs or omega-3s

butter and cream: grass-fed butter and heavy cream

cheese: non-processed cheeses such as cheddar, goat, cream, blue, or mozzarella cheese

nuts and seeds: almonds, walnuts, flaxseeds, pumpkin seeds, chia seeds, etc.

healthy oils: extra virgin olive oil, coconut oil, and avocado oil

avocado: whole avocado or freshly made guacamole

low carb vegetables: green vegetables, tomatoes, onions, peppers, etc.

seasonings: salt, pepper, herbs, and spices

It's best to base your diet primarily on whole, single-ingredient foods. Here's a list of 44 healthy low-carb foods.

Healthy keto snacks

In case you get the urge to eat between meals, here are some healthy, keto-approved snacks:

fatty meat or fish

cheese

a handful of nuts or seeds

keto sushi bites

olives

one or two hard-boiled or deviled eggs

keto-friendly snack bars

90 percent dark chocolate

whole Greek yogurt mixed with nut butter and cocoa powder

peppers and guacamole

strawberries and plain cottage cheese

celery with salsa and guacamole

beef jerky

smaller portions of leftover meals

fat bombs

Keto tips and tricks

Although starting the ketogenic diet can be difficult, there are several tips and tricks you can use to make it easier.

Start by familiarizing yourself with food labels and checking the grams of fat, carbohydrates, and fiber to determine how your favorite foods can fit into your diet.

Planning your meals can also be beneficial and can help you save extra time during the week.

Tips for eating out on a ketogenic diet

Many restaurant meals can be made keto-friendly.

Most restaurants offer some type of meat or fish dish. Order this food and replace any high-carb food with extra vegetables.

Egg meals are also a good option, such as an omelet or eggs and bacon. Another favorite meal is burgers without a bun. You could also replace the fries with veggies. Add extra avocado, cheese, bacon, or eggs.

In Mexican restaurants, you can enjoy any type of meat with extra cheese, guacamole, salsa, and sour cream.

For dessert, ask for a tray of mixed cheeses or berries with cream.

At least, in the beginning, it's crucial to eat until you're full and avoid cutting calories too much. Usually, a ketogenic diet involves weight loss without intentional calorie restriction.

In this Keto cookbook, you can organize your Keto diet with the different dishes you'll find for meals throughout the day. Enjoy!

Breakfast

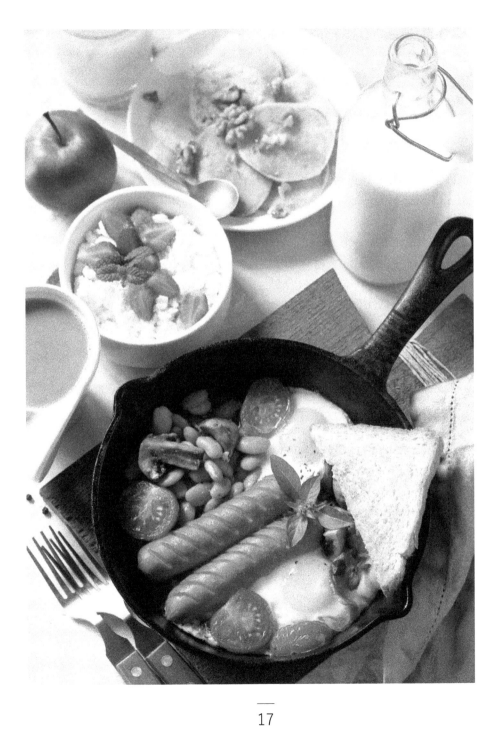

Sage Potato Casserole

Preparation time: 10 minutes
Cooking time: 3 hours and 30 minutes
Servings: 2

Ingredients:
teaspoon onion powder
2 eggs, whisked
½ teaspoon garlic powder
½ teaspoon sage, dried
Salt and black pepper to the taste
½ yellow onion, chopped
tablespoons parsley, chopped
garlic cloves, minced
A pinch of red pepper flakes
½ tablespoon olive oil
2 red potatoes, cubed

Directions:
Grease your slow cooker with the oil, add potatoes, onion, garlic, parsley and pepper flakes and toss a bit.
In a bowl, mix eggs with onion powder, garlic powder, sage, salt and pepper, whisk well and pour over potatoes.
Cover, cook on High for 3 hours and 30 minutes, divide into 2 plates and serve for breakfast.
Enjoy!

Nutrition:
Calories 218, Fat 6, Fiber 6, Carbs 14, Protein 5

Broccoli Casserole

Preparation time: 10 minutes
Cooking time: 6 hours
Servings: 2

Ingredients:
2 eggs, whisked
cup broccoli florets
cups hash browns
½ teaspoon coriander, ground
½ teaspoon rosemary, dried
½ teaspoon turmeric powder
½ teaspoon mustard powder
A pinch of salt and black pepper
1 small red onion, chopped
½ red bell pepper, chopped
1 ounce cheddar cheese, shredded
Cooking spray

Directions:
Grease your slow cooker with the cooking spray, and spread hash browns, broccoli, bell pepper and the onion on the bottom of the pan. In a bowl, mix the eggs with the coriander and the other ingredients, whisk and pour over the broccoli mix in the pot.
Put the lid on, cook on Low for 6 hours, divide between plates and serve for breakfast.

Nutrition:
Calories 261, Fat 7, Fiber 8, Carbs 20, Protein 11

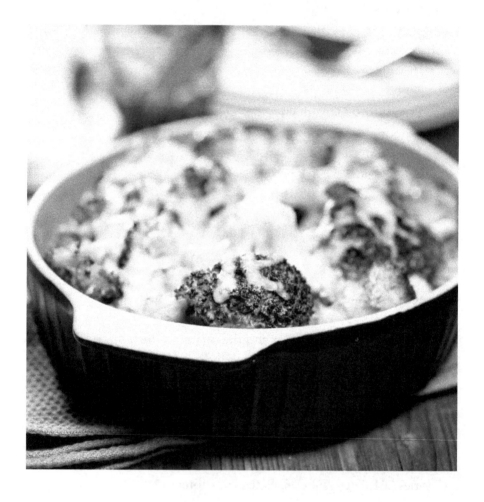

Vegetable Omelet

Preparation time: 10 minutes
Cooking time: 2 hours
Servings: 2

Ingredients:
6 eggs
½ cup milk
¼ teaspoon salt
Black pepper, to taste
1/8 teaspoon garlic powder
1/8 teaspoon chili powder
cup broccoli florets
1 red bell pepper, thinly sliced
1 small yellow onion, finely chopped
1 garlic clove, minced
For Garnishing
Chopped tomatoes
Fresh parsley
Shredded cheddar cheese
Chopped onions

Directions:
Mix together eggs, milk, garlic powder, chili powder, salt and black pepper in a large mixing bowl. Grease a crockpot and add garlic, onions, broccoli florets and sliced peppers. Stir in the egg mixture and cover the lid. Cook on HIGH for about 2 hours. Top with cheese and allow it to stand for about 3 minutes. Dish out the omelet into a serving plate and garnish with chopped onions, chopped tomatoes and fresh parsley.

Nutrition:
Calories 136, Fat 7.4g, Carbohydrates 7.8g

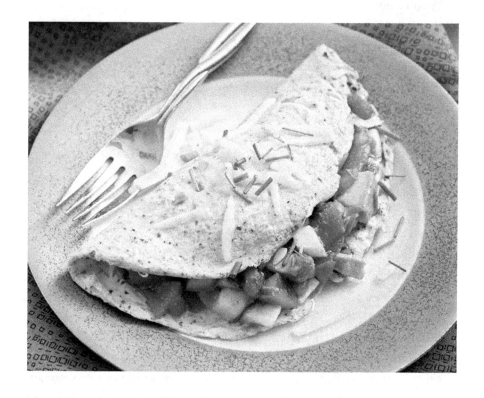

Quinoa and Veggies Casserole

Preparation time: 10 minutes
Cooking time: 6 hours
Servings: 2

Ingredients:
¼ cup quinoa
cup almond milk
eggs, whisked
tablespoon parsley, chopped
1 tablespoon chives, chopped
A pinch of salt and black pepper
¼ cup baby spinach
¼ cup cherry tomatoes, halved
tablespoons parmesan, shredded
Cooking spray

Directions:
Grease your slow cooker with the cooking spray, add the quinoa mixed with the milk, eggs and the other ingredients except the parmesan, toss and spread into the pot. Sprinkle the parmesan on top, put the lid on and cook on Low for 6 hours. Divide between plates and serve.

Nutrition:
Calories 251, Fat 5, Fiber 7, Carbs 19,

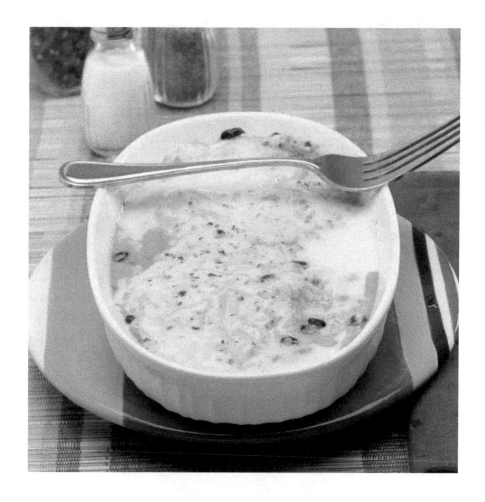

Sausage and Potato Mix

Preparation time: 10 minutes
Cooking time: 6 hours
Servings: 2

Ingredients:
2 sweet potatoes, peeled and roughly cubed
1 green bell pepper, minced
½ yellow onion, chopped
4 ounces smoked Andouille sausage, sliced
1 cup cheddar cheese, shredded
¼ cup Greek yogurt
¼ teaspoon basil, dried
1 cup chicken stock
Salt and black pepper to the taste
1 tablespoon parsley, chopped

Directions:
In your slow cooker, combine the potatoes with the bell pepper, sausage and the other ingredients, toss, put the lid on and cook on Low for 6 hours.
Divide between plates and serve for breakfast.

Nutrition:
Calories 623, Fat 35.7, Fiber 7.6, Carbs 53.1, Protein 24.8

Hash Brown with Bacon

Preparation time: 10 minutes
Cooking time: 3 hours
Servings: 2

Ingredients:
5 ounces hash browns, shredded
2 bacon slices, cooked and chopped
¼ cup mozzarella cheese, shredded
2 eggs, whisked
¼ cup sour cream
tablespoon cilantro, chopped
1 tablespoon olive oil
A pinch of salt and black pepper

Directions:
Grease your slow cooker with the oil, add the hash browns mixed with the eggs, sour cream and the other ingredients, toss, put the lid on and cook on High for 4 hours.
Divide the casserole into bowls and serve.

Nutrition: Calories 383, Fat 26.9, Fiber 2.3, Carbs 26.6, Protein 9.6

Chicken

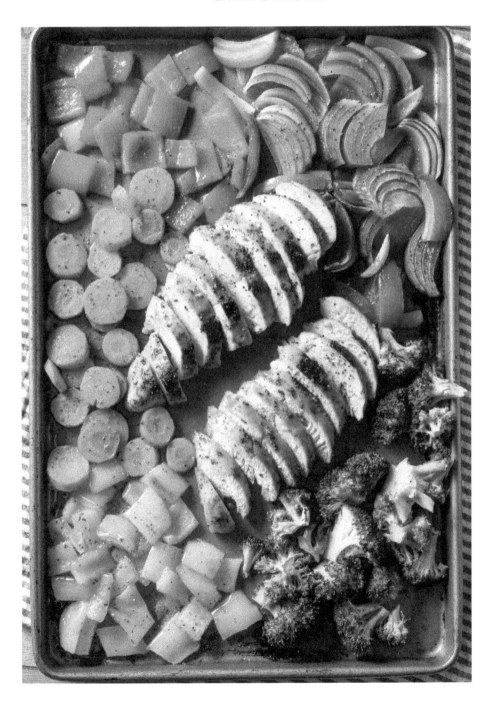

Turkish Chicken Thigh Kebabs

Preparation time: 15 minutes
Cooking time: 9 to 12 minutes
Servings: 2

Ingredients:
1 pound (454 g) chicken thighs, boneless, skinless and halved
½ cup Greek yogurt
Sea salt, to taste
tablespoon Aleppo red pepper flakes
½ teaspoon ground black pepper
¼ teaspoon dried oregano
½ teaspoon mustard seeds
⅛ teaspoon ground cinnamon
½ teaspoon sumac
Roma tomatoes, chopped
2 tablespoons olive oil
1½ ounces (43 g) Swiss cheese, sliced

Directions:
Place the chicken thighs, yogurt, salt, red pepper flakes, black pepper, oregano, mustard seeds, cinnamon, sumac, tomatoes, and olive oil in a ceramic dish. Cover and let it marinate in your refrigerator for 4 hours.
Preheat your grill for medium-high heat and lightly oil the grate.
Thread the chicken thighs onto skewers, making a thick log shape.
Cook your kebabs for 3 or 4 minutes; turn over and continue cooking for 3 to 4 minutes more. An instant-read thermometer should read about 165°F (74°C).
Add the cheese and let it cook for a further 3 to 4 minutes or until completely melted. Bon appétit!

Nutrition:
calories 500, fat 23.3g, protein 61.0g, carbs 6.2g, net carbs 4.5g, fiber 1.7g

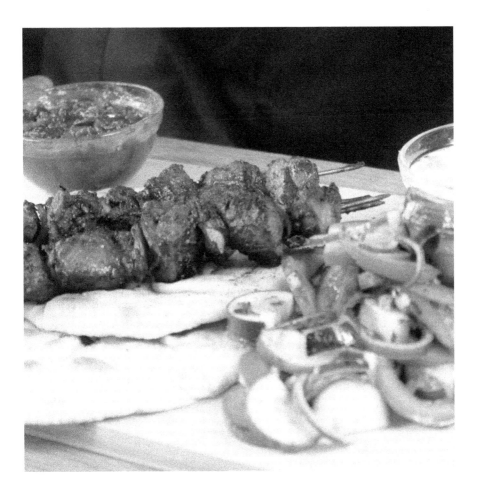

Simple White Wine Drumettes

Preparation time: 10 minutes
Cooking time: 35 minutes
Servings: 4

Ingredients:
1 pound (454 g) chicken drumettes
tablespoon olive oil
tablespoons butter, melted
garlic cloves, sliced
Fresh juice of ½ lemon
tablespoons white wine
Salt and ground black pepper, to taste
1 tablespoon fresh scallions, chopped

Directions:
Start by preheating your oven to 450°F (235°C). Place the chicken in a parchment-lined baking pan. Drizzle with olive oil and melted butter. Add the garlic, lemon, wine, salt, and black pepper.
Bake in the preheated oven for about 35 minutes. Serve garnished with fresh scallions. Enjoy!

Nutrition:
calories 210, fat 12.3g, protein 23.3g, carbs 0.5g, net carbs 0.4g, fiber 0.1g

Chicken Schnitzel

Preparation Time: 15 minutes
Cooking Time: 15-20 minutes
Servings: 4

Ingredients:

1 tbsp. chopped fresh parsley

4 garlic cloves, minced

1 tbsp. plain vinegar

tbsp. coconut aminos

tsp. sugar-free maple syrup

2 tsp. chili pepper

Salt and black pepper to taste

6 tbsp. coconut oil

1 lb. asparagus, stiff stems removed

4 chicken breasts, skin-on and boneless

2 cups grated Mexican cheese blend

1 tbsp. mixed sesame seeds

1 cup almond flour

4 eggs, beaten

6 tbsp. avocado oil

1 tsp. chili flakes for garnish

Directions:

In a bowl, whisk the parsley, garlic, vinegar, coconut aminos, maple syrup, chili pepper, salt, and black pepper. Set aside. Heat the coconut oil in a large skillet and stir-fry the asparagus for 8 to 10 minutes or until tender. Remove the asparagus into a large bowl and toss with the vinegar mixture. Set aside for serving. Cover the chicken breasts in plastic wraps and use a meat tenderizer to pound the chicken until flattened to 2-inch thickness gently. On a plate, mix the Mexican cheese blend and sesame seeds. Dredge the chicken pieces in the almond flour, dip in the egg on both sides, and generously coat in the seed mix. Heat the avocado oil. Cook the chicken until golden brown and cooked within. Divide the asparagus onto four serving plates, place a chicken on each, and garnish with the chili flakes. Serve warm.

Nutrition:

Calories 451, Fat 18.5g, Fiber 12.9g, Carbohydrates 5.9 g, Protein 19.5g

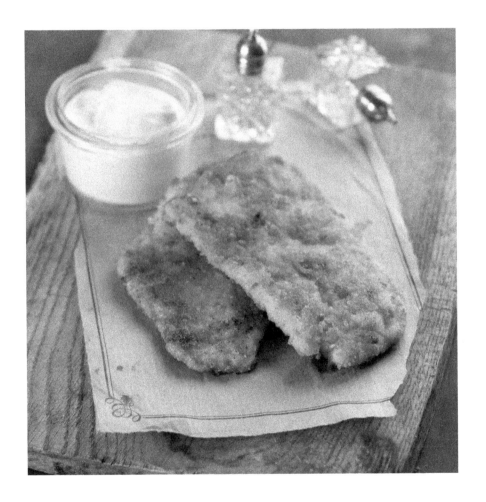

Mediterranean Chicken with Peppers and Olives

Preparation time: 15 minutes
Cooking time: 15 minutes
Servings: 2

Ingredients:
2 chicken drumsticks, boneless and skinless
tablespoon extra-virgin olive oil
Sea salt and ground black pepper, to season
bell peppers, deveined and halved
small chili pepper, finely chopped
tablespoons Greek aioli
6 Kalamata olives, pitted

Directions:
Brush the chicken drumsticks with the olive oil. Season the chicken drumsticks with salt and black pepper.
Preheat your grill to moderate heat. Grill the chicken drumsticks for 8 minutes; turn them over and add the bell peppers.
Grill them for a further 5 minutes. Transfer to a serving platter; top with chopped chili pepper and Greek aioli.
Garnish with Kalamata olives and serve warm. Enjoy!

Nutrition:
calories 400, fat 31.3g, protein 24.5g, carbs 5.0g, net carbs 3.9g, fiber 1.1g

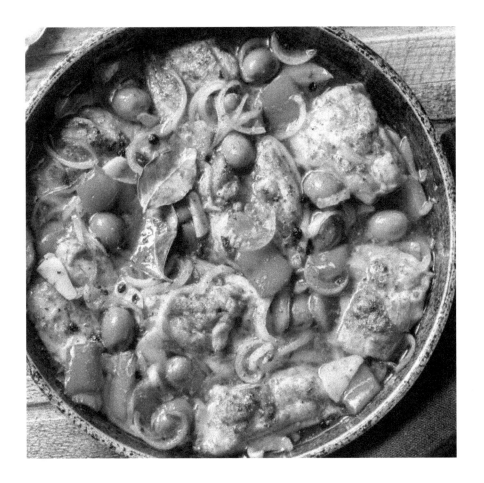

Thai Peanut Chicken Skewers

Preparation Time: 10 minutes
Cooking Time: 15 minutes
Servings: 2

Ingredients:
1-pound boneless skinless chicken breast, cut into chunks
3 tablespoons coconut aminos
1/2 teaspoon Sriracha sauce, plus 1/4 teaspoon
3 teaspoons toasted sesame oil, divided
Ghee, for oiling
2 tablespoons peanut butter
Pink Himalayan salt
Freshly ground black pepper

Directions:
In a bag, combine the chicken chunks with two tablespoons of soy sauce, 1/2 teaspoon of Sriracha sauce, and two teaspoons of sesame oil. Marinate the chicken. If you are using wood 8-inch skewers, soak them in water for 30 minutes before using. Oil the grill pan with ghee. Thread the chicken chunks onto the skewers. Cook the skewers over low heat for 10 to 15 minutes, flipping halfway through. Meanwhile, mix the peanut dipping sauce. Stir together the remaining one tablespoon of soy sauce, 1/4 teaspoon of Sriracha sauce, one teaspoon of sesame oil, and the peanut butter. Season with pink Himalayan salt and pepper. Serve the chicken skewers with a small dish of the peanut sauce.

Nutrition:
Calories 390, Fat 18.4 g, Fiber 12.9g, Carbohydrates 2.1 g, Protein 17.4g

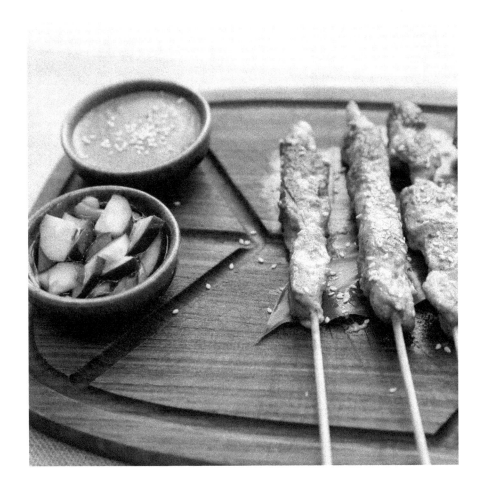

Fried Turkey and Pork Meatballs

Preparation time: 20 minutes
Cooking time: 15 minutes
Servings: 4

Ingredients:
4 spring onions, finely chopped
2 spring garlic stalks, chopped
2 tablespoons cilantro, chopped
½ pound (227 g) ground pork
½ pound (227 g) ground turkey
1 egg, whisked
½ cup Parmesan cheese, grated
teaspoon dried rosemary
½ teaspoon mustard powder
Sea salt and freshly ground black pepper, to season
tablespoons olive oil

Directions:
In a mixing bowl, thoroughly combine all ingredients, except for the olive oil.
Shape the mixture into small balls.
Refrigerate your meatballs for 1 hour.
Then, heat the olive oil in a frying pan over medium-high heat. Once hot, fry
the meatballs for 6 minutes until nicely browned.
Turn them and cook 6 minutes on the other side. Bon appétit!

Nutrition:
calories 367, fat 27.6g, protein 25.9g, carbs 3.0g, net carbs 2.5g, fiber 0.5g

Pork

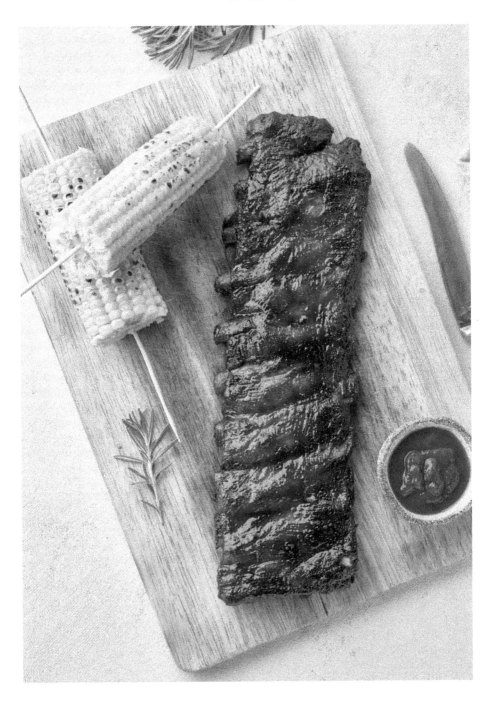

BBQ Pulled Beef

Preparation Time: 15 minutes
Cooking Time: 6 hrs.
Servings: 10

Ingredients:
3 lbs. boneless chuck roast
2 tablespoons of salt
2 tablespoon of garlic powder
tablespoon of onion powder
1/4 apple cider vinegar
tablespoons of coconut aminos
1/2 cup of bone broth
1/4 cup of melted butter
1 tablespoon of black pepper
tablespoon of smoked paprika
tablespoon of tomato paste

Directions:
Mix salt, onion, paprika, black pepper, and garlic. Next is to rub the mixture on the beef and then put the beef in a slow cooker. Use another bowl to melt butter. Then, add a tomato paste, coconut aminos, and vinegar. Pour it all over the beef. Next is to add the bone broth into the slow cooker by pouring it around the beef. Cook for about 6 hrs. After that, take out the beef and increase the temperature of the cooker so that the sauce can thicken. Tear the beef before adding it to the slow cooker and toss with the sauce

Nutrition:
Calories 315, Fat 17g, Fiber 11.9g, Carbohydrates 4.1 g, Protein 18.9g

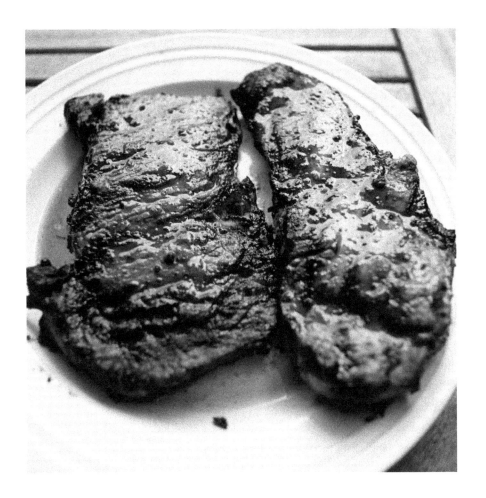

Chili Con Carne

Preparation time: 15 minutes
Cooking time: 45 minutes
Servings: 4

Ingredients:
2 ounces (57 g) bacon, diced
1 red onion, chopped
1 pound (454 g) ground pork
teaspoon ground cumin
cloves garlic, minced
teaspoon chipotle powder
Kosher salt and ground black pepper, to taste
½ cup beef broth
ripe tomatoes, crushed

Directions:
Heat up a medium stockpot over a moderate flame. Cook the bacon until crisp; reserve.

Cook the onion and ground pork in the bacon grease. Cook until the ground pork is no longer pink and the onion just begins to brown.

Stir in the ground cumin and garlic and continue to sauté for 30 seconds more or until aromatic.

Add the chipotle powder, salt, black pepper, broth, and tomatoes to the pot. Cook, partially covered, for 45 minutes or until heated through.

You can add ¼ cup of water during the cooking, as needed. Serve with the reserved bacon and other favorite toppings. Enjoy!

Nutrition:
calories 390, fat 29.8g, protein 22.3g, carbs 5.2g, net carbs 3.7g, fiber 1.5g

Roasted Pork Loin with Brown Mustard Sauce

Preparation Time: 10 minutes
Cooking Time: 70 minutes
Servings: 8

Ingredients:

1 (2-pound) boneless pork loin roast
Sea salt
Freshly ground black pepper
3 tablespoons olive oil
11/2 cups decadent (whipping) cream
3 tablespoons grainy mustard, such as Pommery

Directions:

Preheat the oven to 375°F. Season the pork roast all over with sea salt
and pepper. Heat oil then all the sides of the roast must be browned,
about 6 minutes in total, and place the roast in a baking dish. When
there are approximately 15 minutes of roasting time left, place a small
saucepan over medium heat and add the heavy cream and mustard. Stir
the sauce until it simmers, then reduce the heat to low. Simmer the
sauce until it is vibrant and thick, about 5 minutes. Remove the pan
from the heat and set aside.

Nutrition:

Calories 415, Fat 18.4g, Fiber 11.3g, Carbohydrates 3.1 g,
Protein 17.4g

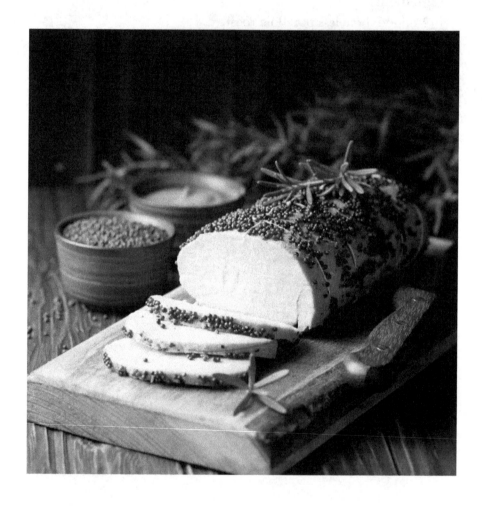

Smoked Sausages with Peppers and Mushrooms

Preparation time: 10 minutes
Cooking time: 1 hour
Servings: 6

Ingredients:

3 yellow bell peppers, seeded and chopped
2 pounds (907 g) smoked sausage, sliced
Salt and black pepper, to taste
2 pounds (907 g) portobello mushrooms, sliced
2 sweet onions, chopped
tablespoon Swerve
tablespoons olive oil
Arugula to garnish

Directions:

In a baking dish, combine the sausages with Swerve, oil, black pepper, onion, bell peppers, salt, and mushrooms. Pour in 1 cup of water and toss well to ensure everything is coated, set in the oven at 320°F (160°C) to bake for 1 hour. To serve, divide the sausages between plates and scatter over the arugula.

Nutrition:

calories 524, fat 32.0g, protein 28.9g, carbs 14.4g, net carbs 7.4g, fiber 7.0g

Pork Cutlets with Juniper Berries

Preparation time: 10 minutes
Cooking time: 20 minutes
Servings: 2

Ingredients:
tablespoon lard, softened at room temperature
pork cutlets, 2-inch-thick
⅓ cup dry red wine
2 garlic cloves, sliced
½ teaspoon whole black peppercorns
4 tablespoons flaky salt
1 teaspoon juniper berries
½ teaspoon cayenne pepper

Directions:
Melt the lard in a nonstick skillet over a moderate flame. Now, brown the pork cutlets for about 8 minutes, turning them over to ensure even cooking; reserve. Add a splash of wine to deglaze the pan. Stir in the remaining ingredients and continue to cook until fragrant or for a minute or so.

Return the pork cutlets to the skillet, continue to cook until the sauce has thickened and everything is heated through about 10 minutes. Serve warm. Bon appétit!

Nutrition:
calories 370, fat 20.5g, protein 40.2g, carbs 1.2g, net carbs 1.0g, fiber 0.2g

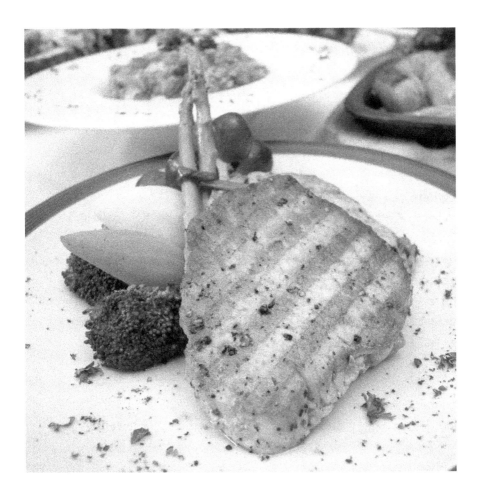

Bacon Smothered Pork with Thyme

Preparation time: 10 minutes
Cooking time: 20 minutes
Servings: 6

Ingredients:

7 strips bacon, chopped
6 pork chops
Pink salt and black pepper to taste
5 sprigs fresh thyme plus extra to garnish
¼ cup chicken broth
½ cup heavy cream

Directions:

Cook bacon in a large skillet on medium heat for 5 minutes. Remove with a slotted spoon onto a paper towel-lined plate to soak up excess fat.

Season pork chops with salt and black pepper, and brown in the bacon fat for 4 minutes on each side. Remove to the bacon plate. Stir in the thyme, chicken broth, and heavy cream and simmer for 5 minutes.

Return the chops and bacon, and cook further for another 2 minutes. Serve chops and a generous ladle of sauce with cauli mash. Garnish with thyme leaves.

Nutrition:

calories 434, fat 37.1g, protein 22.1g, carbs 3.1g, net carbs 2.9g, fiber 0.2g

Beef and Lamb

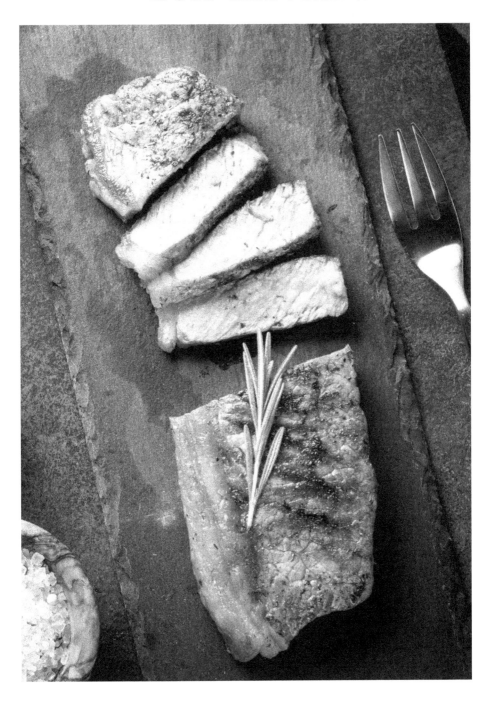

Butternut Squash and Beef Stew

Preparation time: 15 minutes
Cooking time: 35 minutes
Servings: 4

Ingredients:
3 teaspoons olive oil
1 pound (454 g) ground beef
1 cup beef stock
14 ounces (397 g) canned tomatoes with juice
1 tablespoon stevia
1 pound (454 g) butternut squash, chopped
tablespoon Worcestershire sauce
bay leaves
Salt and black pepper, to taste
1 onion, chopped
1 teaspoon dried sage
1 tablespoon garlic, minced

Directions:
Set a pan over medium heat and heat olive oil, stir in the onion, garlic, and beef, and cook for 10 minutes. Add in butternut squash, Worcestershire sauce, bay leaves, stevia, beef stock, canned tomatoes, and sage, and bring to a boil. Reduce heat, and simmer for 30 minutes.
Remove and discard the bay leaves and adjust the seasonings. Split into bowls and enjoy.

Nutrition:
calories 342, fat 17.1g, protein 31.9g, carbs 11.6g, net carbs 7.4g, fiber 4.2g

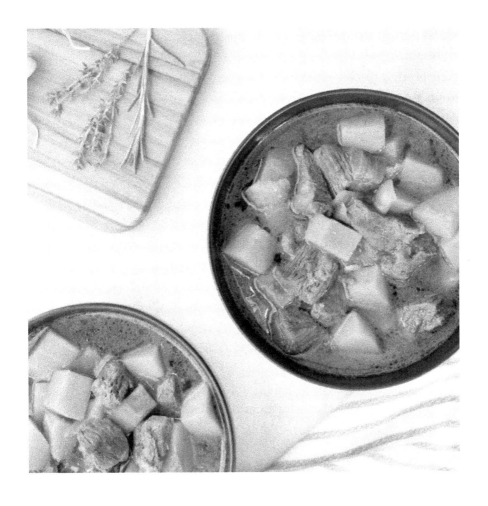

Braised Beef Chuck Roast with Tomatoes

Preparation time: 15 minutes
Cooking time: 7 to 8 hours
Servings: 4

Ingredients:

3 tablespoons extra-virgin olive oil, divided
1 pound (454 g) beef chuck roast, cut into 1-inch cubes
Salt, for seasoning
Freshly ground black pepper, for seasoning
(15-ounce / 425-g) can diced tomatoes
tablespoons tomato paste
2 teaspoons minced garlic
2 teaspoons dried basil
1 teaspoon dried oregano
½ teaspoon whole black peppercorns
cup shredded Mozzarella cheese, for garnish
tablespoons chopped parsley, for garnish

Directions:

Lightly grease the insert of the slow cooker with 1 tablespoon of the
olive oil.
In a large skillet over medium-high heat, heat the remaining 2
tablespoons of the olive oil. Season the beef with salt and pepper. Add
the beef to the sillet and brown for 7 minutes. Transfer the beef to the
insert. In a medium bowl, stir together the tomatoes, tomato paste,
garlic, basil, oregano, and peppercorns, and add the tomato mixture to
the beef in the insert.
Cover and cook on low for 7 to 8 hours. Serve topped with the cheese
and parsley.

Nutrition:

calories 540, fat 42.9g, protein 29.8g, carbs 6.9g, net carbs 4.8g,
fiber 2.1g

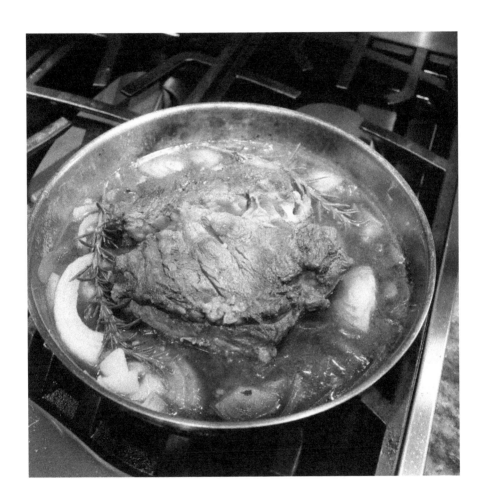

Sour Cream Beef Carne Asada

Preparation time: 15 minutes
Cooking time: 9 to 10 hours
Servings: 8

Ingredients:
½ cup extra-virgin olive oil, divided
¼ cup lime juice
2 tablespoons apple cider vinegar
2 teaspoons minced garlic
1½ teaspoons paprika
1 teaspoon ground cumin
1 teaspoon chili powder
¼ teaspoon cayenne pepper
sweet onion, cut into eighths
pounds (907 g) beef rump roast
1 cup sour cream, for garnish

Directions:
Lightly grease the insert of the slow cooker with 1 tablespoon of the olive oil.
In a small bowl, whisk together the remaining olive oil, lime juice, apple cider vinegar, garlic, paprika, cumin, chili powder, and cayenne until well blended.
Place the onion in the bottom of the insert and the beef on top of the vegetable. Pour the sauce over the beef.
Cover and cook on low for 9 to 10 hours.
Shred the beef with a fork.
Serve topped with the sour cream.

Nutrition:
calories 540, fat 43.9g, protein 30.9g, carbs 2.9g, net carbs 1.9g, fiber 1.0g

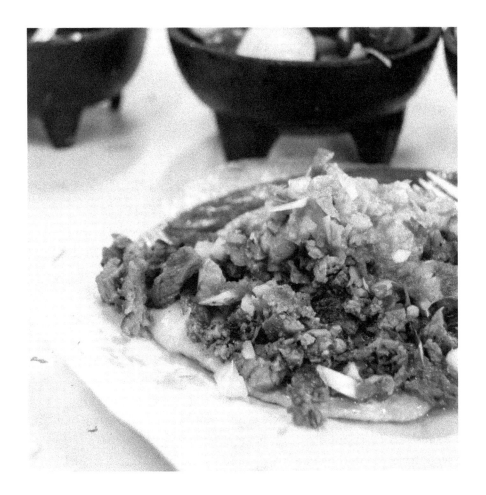

Balsamic Skirt Steak

Prep time: 2 minutes
Cooking time: 6 minutes
Servings: 6

Ingredients:
¼ cup balsamic vinegar (no sugar added)
2 tablespoons extra-virgin olive oil
1 tablespoon fresh chopped parsley
1 teaspoon minced garlic
teaspoon kosher salt
¼ teaspoon ground black pepper
pounds (907 g) skirt steak, trimmed of fat

Directions:
In a medium-sized bowl, whisk together the vinegar, olive oil, parsley, garlic, salt, and pepper. Add the skirt steak and flip to ensure that the entire surface is covered in marinade. Cover with plastic wrap and marinate in the refrigerator for at least 2 hours, or up to 24 hours.
Take the bowl out of the refrigerator and let the steak and marinade come to room temperature. Meanwhile, preheat a grill to high heat. Remove the steak from the marinade (reserve the marinade) and place on the grill over direct high heat. Grill for 3 minutes per side for medium (recommended) or 5 minutes per side for well-done.
Remove the steak from the grill when the desired doneness is reached and let rest for 10 minutes before slicing. Meanwhile, place the reserved marinade in the microwave and cook on high for 3 minutes, or until boiling. Stir and set aside; you will use the boiled marinade as a sauce for the steak.
Slice the steak, being sure to cut against the grain for best results. Serve with the sauce.
Nutrition:
calories 355, fat 25.1g, protein 30.9g, carbs 0g, net carbs 0g, fiber 0

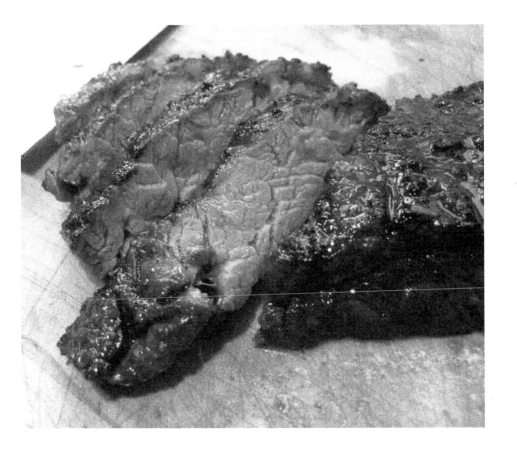

Beef and Fennel Provençal

Preparation time: 10 minutes
Cooking time: 45 minutes
Servings: 4

Ingredients:
12 ounces (340 g) beef steak racks
fennel bulbs, sliced
Salt and black pepper, to taste
tablespoons olive oil
½ cup apple cider vinegar
1 teaspoon herbs de Provence
1 tablespoon Swerve

Directions:
In a bowl, mix the fennel with 2 tablespoons of oil, Swerve, and vinegar, toss to coat well, and set to a baking dish. Season with herbs de Provence, pepper and salt, and cook in the oven at 400°F (205°C)
for 15 minutes.
Sprinkle black pepper and salt to the beef, place into an oiled pan over medium heat, and cook for a couple of minutes. Place the beef to the baking dish with the fennel, and bake for 20 minutes. Split everything among plates and enjoy.

Nutrition:
calories 231, fat 11.4g, protein 19.1g, carbs 8.7g, net carbs 5.1g, fiber 3.6g

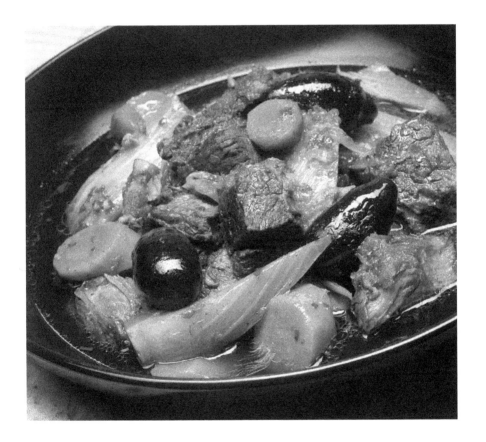

Beef and Cauliflower Stuffed Peppers

Preparation time: 25 minutes
Cooking time: 6 hours
Servings: 4

Ingredients:
3 tablespoons extra-virgin olive oil, divided
1 pound (454 g) ground beef
½ cup finely chopped cauliflower
tomato, diced
½ sweet onion, chopped
teaspoons minced garlic
2 teaspoons dried oregano
1 teaspoon dried basil
4 bell peppers, tops cut off and seeded
1 cup shredded Cheddar cheese
½ cup chicken broth
1 tablespoon basil, sliced into thin strips, for garnish

Directions:
Lightly grease the insert of the slow cooker with 1 tablespoon of the olive oil. In a large skillet over medium-high heat, heat the remaining 2 tablespoons of the olive oil. Add the beef and sauté until it is cooked through, about 10 minutes. Add the cauliflower, tomato, onion, garlic, oregano, and basil. Sauté for an additional 5 minutes.
Spoon the meat mixture into the bell peppers and top with the cheese. Place the peppers in the slow cooker and add the broth to the bottom. Cover and cook on low for 6 hours.
Serve warm, topped with the basil.

Nutrition:
calories 572, fat 41.1g, protein 38.2g, carbs 11.9g, net carbs 8.8g, fiber 3.1g

Fish and Seafood

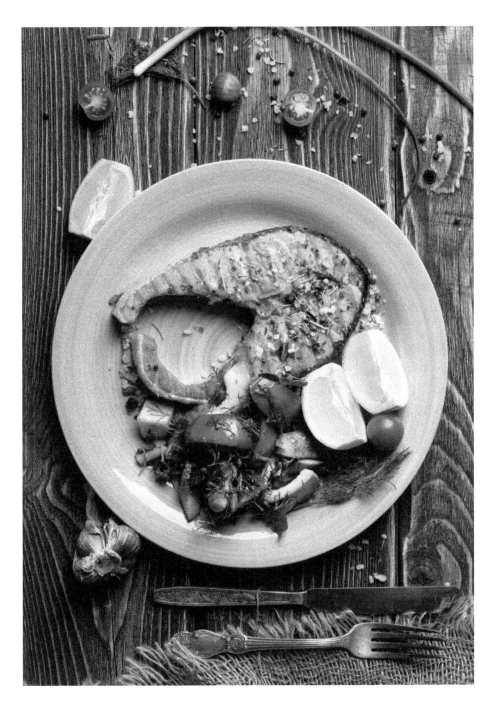

BLT Salad

Preparation Time: 15 minutes
Cooking Time: 0 minutes
Servings: 4

Ingredients:
2 tablespoons melted bacon fat
2 tablespoons red wine vinegar
Freshly ground black pepper
4 cups shredded lettuce
1 tomato, chopped
6 bacon slices, cooked and chopped
2 hardboiled eggs, chopped
1 tablespoon roasted unsalted sunflower seeds
1 teaspoon toasted sesame seeds
1 cooked chicken breast, sliced (optional)

Directions:
In a medium bowl, whisk together the bacon fat and vinegar until emulsified. Season with black pepper. Add the tomato and lettuce to the bowl and toss the vegetables with the dressing. Divide the salad between 4 plates and top each with equal amounts of bacon, egg, sunflower seeds, sesame seeds, and chicken (if using). Serve.

Nutrition:
Calories 287, Fat 9.4g, Fiber 11g, Carbohydrates 3.8 g, Protein 9.9g

Creamy Shrimp

Preparation Time: 10 minutes
Cooking Time: 2 hours 10 minutes
Servins: 4

Ingredients:
1 lb. cooked shrimp
1 cup sour cream
10.5oz. can cream of mushroom soup
1tsp. curry powder
1 onion, chopped

Directions:
Spray a medium pan with cooking spray and heat over medium heat.
Add onion to the hot pan and sauté until onion is soft.
Transfer sautéed onion to a crock pot along with the shrimp, curry powder, and cream of mushroom soup.
Cover and cook on low for 2 hours.
Stir in sour cream and serve.

Nutrition:
Calories 302, Fat 16.2 g, Carbohydrates 9.5 g, Sugar 1.8 g, Protein 28.6 g, Cholesterol 264 mg

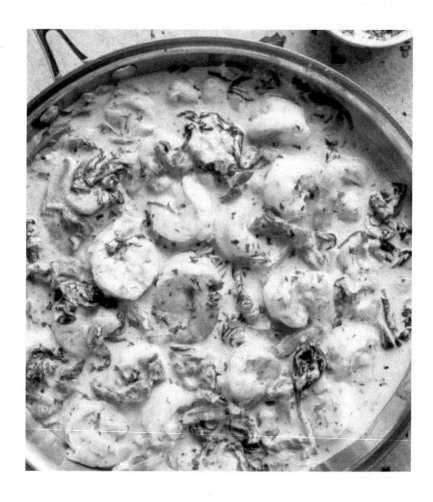

Lemon Trout

Preparation time: 15 minutes
Cooking time: 5 hours
Servings: 4

Ingredients:

1-pound trout, peeled, cleaned
1 lemon, sliced
1 teaspoon dried thyme
1 teaspoon ground black pepper
1 tablespoon olive oil
½ teaspoon salt
½ cup of water

Directions:

Rub the fish with dried thyme, ground black pepper, and salt.
Then fill the fish with sliced lemon and sprinkle with olive oil.
Place the trout in the slow cooker and add water.
Cook the fish on Low for 5 hours.

Nutrition:

252 calories, 30.4g protein, 1.9g carbohydrates, 13.2g fat, 0.6g fiber, 84mg cholesterol, 368mg sodium, 554mg potassium.

Avocado and Prosciutto Deviled Eggs

Preparation Time: 20 minutes
Cooking Time: 10 minutes
Servings: 4

Ingredients:
4 eggs
Ice bath
4 prosciutto slices, chopped
1 avocado, pitted and peeled
1 tbsp. mustard
1 tsp. plain vinegar
1 tbsp. heavy cream
1 tbsp. chopped fresh cilantro
Salt and black pepper to taste
1/2 cup (113 g) mayonnaise
1 tbsp. coconut cream
1/4 tsp. cayenne pepper
1 tbsp. avocado oil
1 tbsp. chopped fresh parsley

Directions:

Boil the eggs for 8 minutes. Remove the eggs into the ice bath, sit for 3 minutes, and then peel the eggs. Slice the eggs lengthwise into halves and empty the egg yolks into a bowl. Arrange the egg whites on a plate with the hole side facing upwards. While the eggs are cooked, heat a non-stick skillet over medium heat and cook the prosciutto for 5 to 8 minutes. Remove the prosciutto onto a paper towel-lined plate to drain grease. Put the avocado slices to the egg yolks and mash both ingredients with a fork until smooth. Mix in the mustard, vinegar, heavy cream, cilantro, salt, and black pepper until well-blended. Spoon the mixture into a piping bag and press the mixture into the egg holes until well-filled. In a bowl, whisk the mayonnaise, coconut cream, cayenne pepper, and avocado oil. On serving plates, spoon some of the mayonnaise sauce and slightly smear it in a circular movement. Top with the deviled eggs, scatter the prosciutto on top and garnish with the parsley. Enjoy immediately.

Nutrition:

Calories 265, Fat 11.7g, Fiber 4.1g, Carbohydrates 3.1 g, Protein 7.9 g

Salmon Croquettes

Preparation time: 10 minutes
Cooking time: 2 hours
Servings: 4

Ingredients:
1-pound salmon fillet, minced
tablespoon mayonnaise
tablespoons panko breadcrumbs
½ teaspoon ground black pepper
1 egg, beaten
1 teaspoon smoked paprika
½ cup of water

Directions:
In the bowl mix minced salmon with mayonnaise panko breadcrumbs, ground black pepper, egg, and smoked paprika. Then make the small croquettes and place them in the slow cooker. Add water and close the lid. Cook the meal on high for 2 hours.

Nutrition:
127 calories, 5.9g protein, 2.2g carbohydrates, 6.3g fat, 0.4g fiber, 61mg cholesterol, 73mg sodium, 311mg potassium.

Salmon with Radish and Arugula Salad

Preparation time: 15 minutes
Cooking time: 10 minutes
Servings: 4

Ingredients:
1 pound (454 g) salmon, cut into 4 steaks each
1 cup radishes, sliced
Salt and black pepper to taste
8 green olives, pitted and chopped
cup arugula
large tomatoes, diced
tablespoons red wine vinegar
green onions, sliced
tablespoons olive oil
2 slices zero carb bread, cubed
¼ cup parsley, chopped

Directions:
In a bowl, mix the radishes, olives, black pepper, arugula, tomatoes, wine vinegar, green onion, olive oil, bread, and parsley. Let sit for the flavors to incorporate. Season the salmon steaks with salt and pepper; grill on both sides for 8 minutes in total. Serve the salmon on a bed of the radish salad.

Nutrition:
calories 339, fat 21.6g, protein 28.4g, carbs 5.3g, net carbs 3.0g, fiber 2.3g

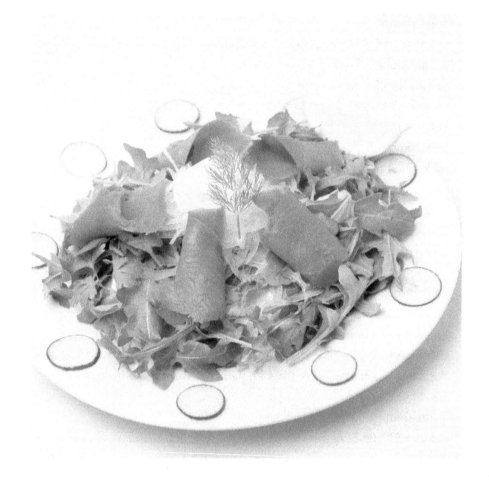

Soups

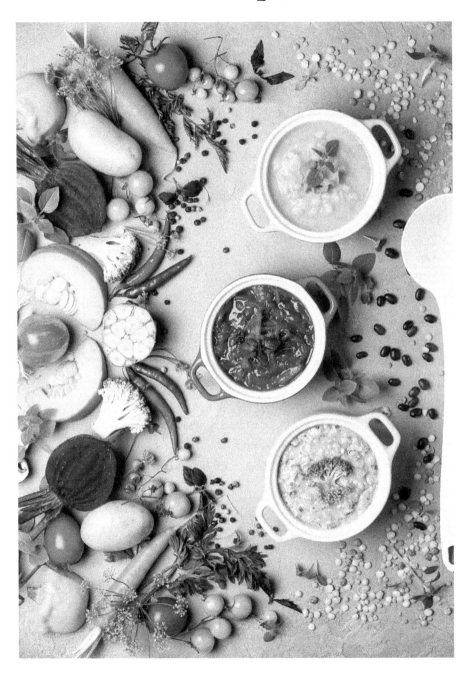

Cream of Broccoli Soup

Preparation time: 15 minutes
Cookings time: 20 minutes
Servings: 4

Ingredients:

3 tablespoons olive oil
1 celery rib, chopped
½ white onion, finely chopped
1 teaspoon ginger-garlic paste
1 (1-pound / 454-g) head broccoli, broken into florets
4 cups vegetable broth
½ cup double cream
1½ cups Monterey Jack cheese, grated

Directions:

Heat the olive oil in a soup pot over moderate heat. Now, sauté the celery rib and onion until they have softened.

Fold in the ginger-garlic paste and broccoli; pour in the vegetable broth and bring to boil. Turn the heat to simmer. Continue to cook for a further 13 minutes or until the broccoli is cooked through.

Fold in the cream, stir and remove from heat. Divide your soup between four ramekins and top them with the Monterey Jack cheese.

Broil for about 5 minutes or until cheese is bubbly and golden. Bon appétit!

Nutrition:

calories 324, fat 28.1g, protein 13.3g, carbs 4.3g, net carbs 3.8g, fiber 0.5g

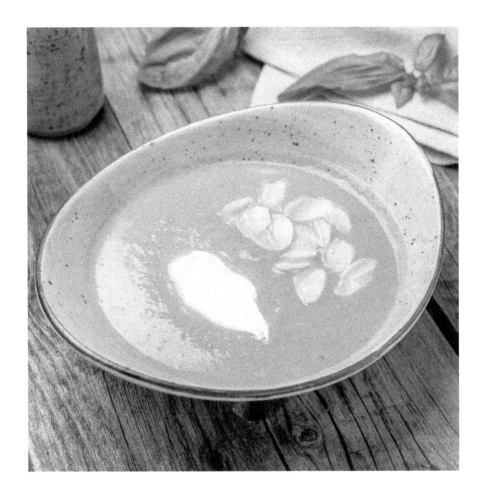

Lobster Soup

Preparation time: 10 minutes
Cooking time: 2. Hours
Servings: 4

Ingredients:
4 cups of water
1-pound lobster tail, chopped
½ cup fresh cilantro, chopped
1 cup coconut cream
1 teaspoon ground coriander
1 garlic clove, diced

Directions:
Pour water and coconut cream in the slow cooker.
Add a lobster tail, cilantro, and ground coriander.
Then add the garlic clove and close the lid.
Cook the lobster soup on High for 2 hours.

Nutrition:
241 calories, 23g protein, 3.6g carbohydrates, 15.2g fat, 1.4g fiber, 165mg cholesterol, 568mg sodium, 435mg potassium

Chicken and Noodles Soup

Preparation time: 10 minutes
Cooking time: 7 hours
Servings: 8

Ingredients:
1-pound chicken breast, skinless, boneless, chopped
1 teaspoon salt
1 teaspoon chili flakes
1 teaspoon coriander
1 cup bell pepper, chopped
4 oz. egg noodles 8 cups chicken stock

Directions:
Mix chicken breast with salt, chili flakes, coriander, and place in the slow cooker.
Add chicken stock and close the lid.
Cook the ingredients on Low for 6 hours.
Then add egg noodles and bell pepper and cook the soup for 1 hour on High.

Nutrition:
99 calories, 13.5g protein, 5.4g carbohydrates, 2.3g fat, 0.4g fiber,
40mg cholesterol, 1084mg sodium, 259mg potassium

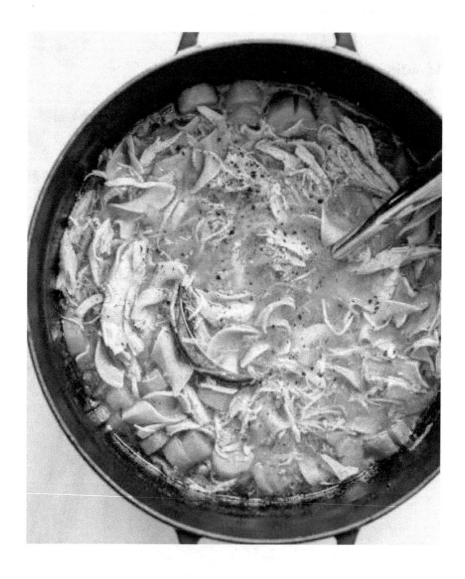

Shrimp Chowder

Preparation time: 5 minutes
Cooking time: 1 hours
Servings: 4

Ingredients:
1-pound shrimps
½ cup fennel bulb, chopped
1 bay leaf
½ teaspoon teaspoon peppercorn
1 cup of coconut milk
3 cups of water
1 ground coriander

Directions:
Put all ingredients in the slow cooker.
Close the lid and cook the chowder on High for 1 hour.

Nutrition:
277 calories, 27.4g protein, 6.1g carbohydrates, 16.3g fat, 1.8g fiber, 239mg cholesterol, 297mg sodium, 401mg potassium

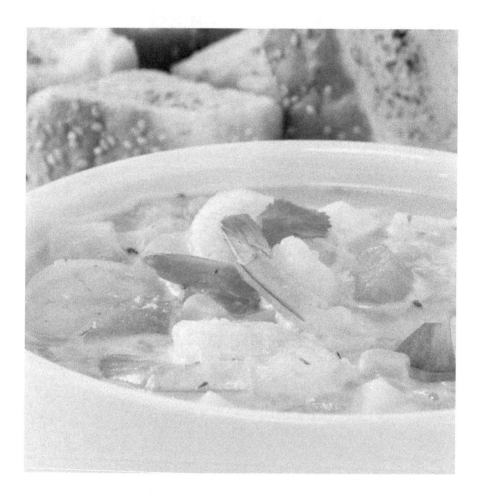

Pork and Mustard Green Soup

Preparation time: 15 minutes
Cooking time: 20 minutes
Servings: 2

Ingredients:
1 tablespoon olive oil
bell pepper, deveined and chopped
garlic cloves, pressed
½ cup scallions, chopped
½ pound (227 g) ground pork (84% lean)
1 cup beef bone broth
1 cup water
½ teaspoon crushed red pepper flakes
Sea salt and freshly cracked black pepper, to season
1 bay laurel
teaspoon fish sauce
cups mustard greens, torn into pieces
1 tablespoon fresh parsley, chopped

Directions:
Heat the olive oil in a stockpot over a moderate flame. Coat, once hot, sauté the pepper, garlic, and scallions until tender or about 3 minutes. After that, stir in the ground pork and cook for 5 minutes more or until well browned, stirring periodically.

Add in the beef bone broth, water, red pepper, salt, black pepper, and bay laurel. Reduce the temperature to simmer and cook, covered, for 10 minutes. Afterwards, stir in the fish sauce and mustard greens. Remove from the heat; let it stand until the greens are wilted. Ladle into individual bowls and serve garnished with fresh parsley.

Nutrition:
calories 345, fat 25.1g, protein 23.2g, carbs 6.2g, net carbs 3.2g, fiber 3.0g

White Mushroom Soup

Preparation time: 15 minutes
Cooking time: 8 hours
Servings: 6

Ingredients:
9 oz. white mushrooms, chopped
6 chicken stock
1 teaspoon dried cilantro
½ teaspoon ground black pepper
1 teaspoon butter
1 cup potatoes, chopped
½ carrot, diced

Directions:
Melt butter in the skillet.
Add white mushrooms and roast them for 5 minutes on high heat. Stir the mushrooms constantly.
Transfer them in the slow cooker.
Add chicken stock, cilantro, ground black pepper, and potato.
Add carrot and close the lid.
Cook the soup on low for 8 hours.

Nutrition:
44 calories, 2.5g protein, 6.7g carbohydrates, 1.4g fat, 1.2g fiber, 2mg cholesterol, 776mg sodium, 271mg potassium

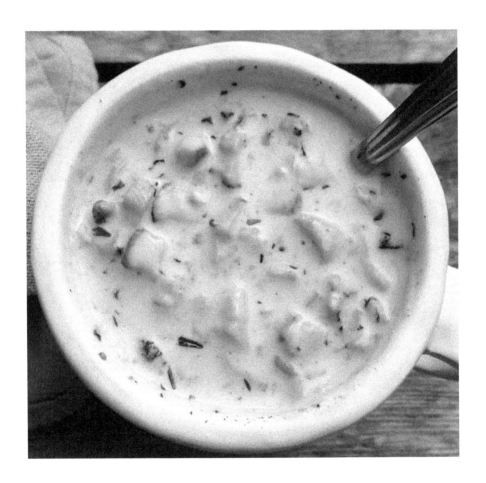

Snacks and Appetizer

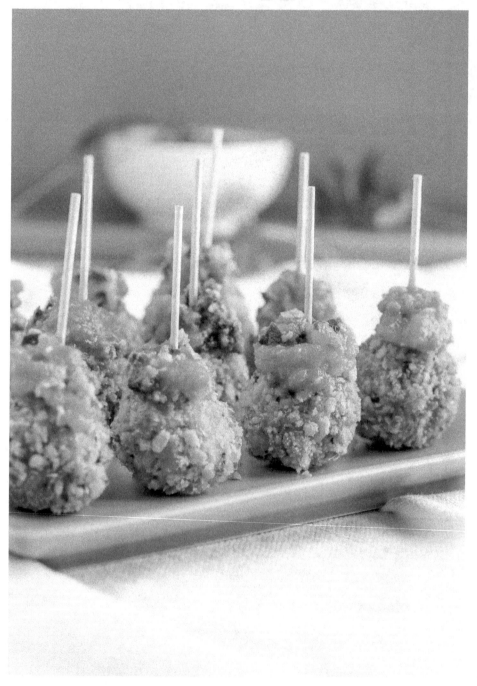

Bacon-Wrapped Poblano Poppers

Preparation time: 15 minutes
Cook time: 30 minutes
Servings: 16

Ingredients:

10 ounces (283 g) cottage cheese, at room temperature

6 ounces (170 g) Swiss cheese, shredded

Sea salt and ground black pepper, to taste

½ teaspoon shallot powder

½ teaspoon cumin powder

⅓ teaspoon mustard seeds

16 poblano peppers, deveined and halved

16 thin slices bacon, sliced lengthwise

Directions:

Mix the cheese, salt, black pepper, shallot powder, cumin, and mustard seeds until well combined.

Divide the mixture between the pepper halves. Wrap each pepper with 2 slices of bacon; secure with toothpicks.

Arrange the stuffed peppers on the rack in the baking sheet.

Bake in the preheated oven at 390°F (199°C) for about 30 minutes until the bacon is sizzling and browned. Bon appétit!

Nutrition:

calories 184, fat 14.1g, protein 8.9g, carbs 5.8g, net carbs 5.0g, fiber 0.8g

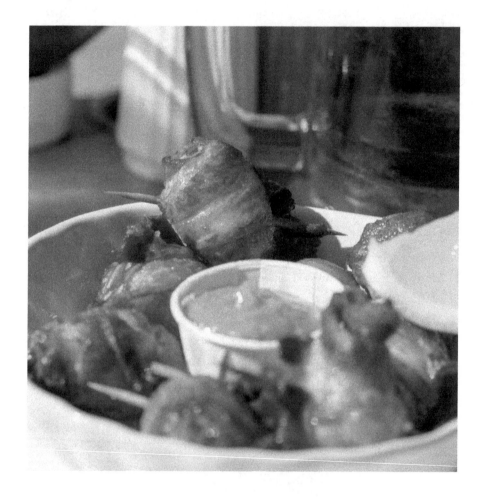

Spinach Spread

Preparation time: 10 minutes
Cooking time: 2 hours
Servings: 2

Ingredients:
4 ounces baby spinach
2 tablespoons mayonnaise
2 ounces heavy cream
½ teaspoon turmeric powder
A pinch of salt and black pepper
ounce Swiss cheese, shredded

Directions:
In your slow cooker, mix the spinach with the cream, mayo and the other ingredients, toss, put the lid on and cook on Low for 2 hours.
Divide into bowls and serve as a party spread.

Nutrition
Calories 132, Fat 4, Fiber 3, Carbs 10, Protein 4

Blueberry Fat Bombs

Preparation Time: 10 minutes
Cooking Time: 0 minutes
Servings: 12

Ingredients:
1/2 cup blueberries, mashed
1/2 cup coconut oil, at room temperature
1/2 cup cream cheese, at room temperature
1 pinch nutmeg
6 drops liquid stevia

Directions:
Line the 12-cup muffin tin with 12 paper liners.
Put all the ingredients and process until it has a thick and mousse-like consistency.
Pour the mixture into the 12 cups of the muffin tin. Put the muffin tin into the refrigerate to chill for 1 to 3 hours.

Nutrition:
Calories 120, Fat 12.5g, Fiber 1.4g, Carbohydrates 2.1 g, Protein 3.1 g

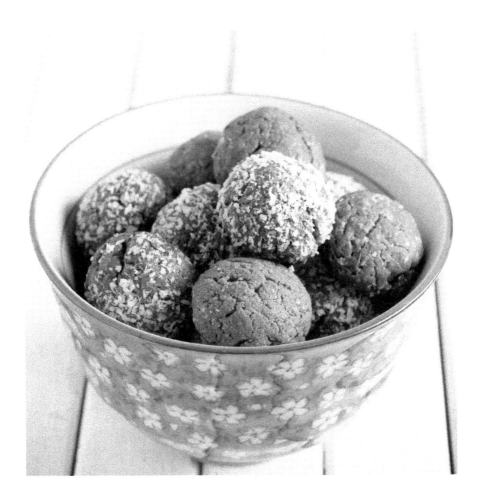

Squash Salsa

Preparation time: 10 minutes
Cooking time: 3 hours
Servings: 2

Ingredients:
1 cup butternut squash, peeled and cubed
1 cup cherry tomatoes, cubed
1 cup avocado, peeled, pitted and cubed
½ tablespoon balsamic vinegar
½ tablespoon lemon juice
1 tablespoon lemon zest, grated
¼ cup veggie stock
1 tablespoon chives, chopped
A pinch of rosemary, dried
A pinch of sage, dried
A pinch of salt and black pepper

Directions:
In your slow cooker, mix the squash with the tomatoes, avocado and the other ingredients, toss, put the lid on and cook on Low for 3 hours. Divide into bowls and serve as a snack.

Nutrition:
Calories 182, Fat 5, Fiber 7, Carbs 12, Protein 5

Anchovy Fat Bombs

Preparation time: 15 minutes
Cooking time: 0 minutes
Servings: 10

Ingredients:

8 ounces (227 g) Cheddar cheese, shredded
6 ounces (170 g) cream cheese, at room temperature
4 ounces (113 g) canned anchovies, chopped
½ yellow onion, minced
1 teaspoon fresh garlic, minced
Sea salt and ground black pepper, to taste

Directions:

Mix all of the above ingredients in a bowl. Place the mixture in your refrigerator for 1 hour.
Then, shape the mixture into bite-sized balls.
Serve immediately.

Nutrition:

calories 123, fat 8.8g, protein 7.4g, carbs 3.3g, net carbs 3.3g, fiber 0g

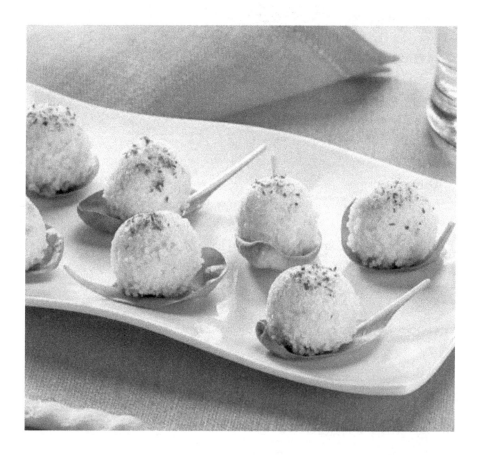

Fried Chicken Strips

Preparation time: 15 minutes
Cooking time: 10 minutes
Servings: 4

Ingredients:

3 tablespoons olive oil
pound (454 g) chicken breasts, sliced
1¼ cups mayonnaise
¼ cup coconut flour
eggs
Salt and black pepper to taste
1 cup Cheddar cheese, grated
4 tablespoons mint, chopped
1 cup Greek yogurt
1 teaspoon garlic powder
tablespoon chopped parsley
green onions, chopped

Directions:

First make the dip: in a bowl, mix 1 cup of the mayonnaise, 3 tablespoons of mint, yogurt, garlic powder, green onion, and salt. Cover the bowl with plastic wrap and refrigerate for 30 minutes. Mix the chicken, remaining mayonnaise, coconut flour, eggs, salt, black pepper, Cheddar cheese, and remaining mint, in a bowl. Cover the bowl with plastic wrap and refrigerate it for 2 hours. Place a skillet over medium heat to warm the olive oil. Fetch 2 tablespoons of chicken mixture into the skillet, use the back of a spatula to flatten the top. Cook for 4 minutes, flip, and fry for 4 minutes more. Remove onto a wire rack and repeat the cooking process until the batter is finished, adding more oil as needed. Garnish the fritters with parsley and serve with mint dip.

Nutrition: calories 673, fat 56.9g, protein 32.1g, carbs 8.6g, net carbs 6.6g, fiber 2.0g

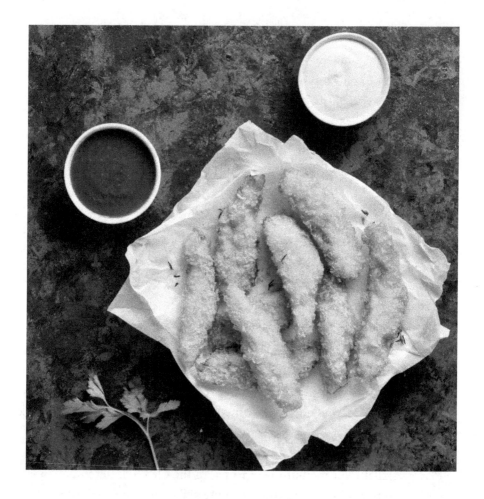

Dessert

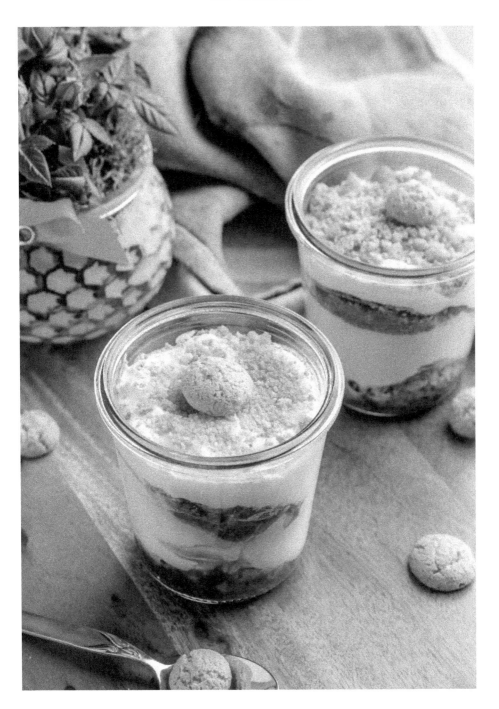

Chocolate Pudding

Preparation Time: 15 minutes
Cooking Time: 45 minutes
Servings: 2

Ingredients:
1/2 teaspoon stevia powder
2 tablespoons cocoa powder
2 tablespoons water
1 tablespoon gelatin
1 cup of coconut milk
2 tablespoons maple syrup

Directions:
Heat pan with the coconut milk over medium heat; add stevia and cocoa powder and mix well.
In a bowl, mix gelatin with water; stir well and add to the pan.
Stir well, add maple syrup, whisk again, divide into ramekins and keep in the fridge for 45 minutes. Serve cold.

Nutrition:
Calories 287, Fat 10.4g, Fiber 9g, Carbohydrates 2.1 g, Protein 3.1g

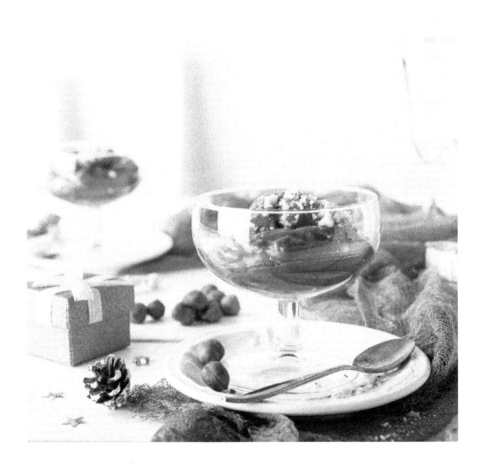

Dates and Rice Pudding

Preparation time: 10 minutes
Cooking time: 3 hours
Servings: 2

Ingredients:
cup dates, chopped
½ cup white rice
cup almond milk
tablespoons brown sugar
1 teaspoon almond extract

Directions:
In your slow cooker, mix the rice with the milk and the other ingredients, whisk, put the lid on and cook on Low for 3 hours.
Divide the pudding into bowls and serve.

Nutrition:
Calories 152, Fat 5, Fiber 2, Carb 6, Protein 3

Apple, Avocado and Mango Bowls

Preparation time: 10 minutes
Cooking time: 2 hours
Servings: 2

Ingredients:
cup avocado, peeled, pitted and cubed
1 cup mango, peeled and cubed
apple, cored and cubed
tablespoons brown sugar
1 cup heavy cream
1 tablespoon lemon juice

Directions:
In your slow cooker, combine the avocado with the mango and the other ingredients, toss gently, put the lid on and cook on Low for 2 hours.
Divide the mix into bowls and serve.

Nutrition:
Calories 60, Fat 1, Fiber 2, Carbs 20, Protein 1

Greek Cream Cheese Pudding

Preparation time: 5 minutes
Cooking time: 2 hours
Servings: 2

Ingredients:
cup cream cheese, soft
½ cup Greek yogurt
eggs, whisked
½ teaspoon baking soda
1 cup almonds, chopped
1 tablespoon sugar
½ teaspoon almond extract
½ teaspoon cinnamon powder

Directions:
In your slow cooker, mix the cream cheese with the yogurt, eggs and the other ingredients, whisk, put the lid on and cook on Low for 2 hours.
Divide the pudding into bowls and serve.

Nutrition:
Calories 172, Fat 2, Fiber 3, Carbs 4, Protein 5

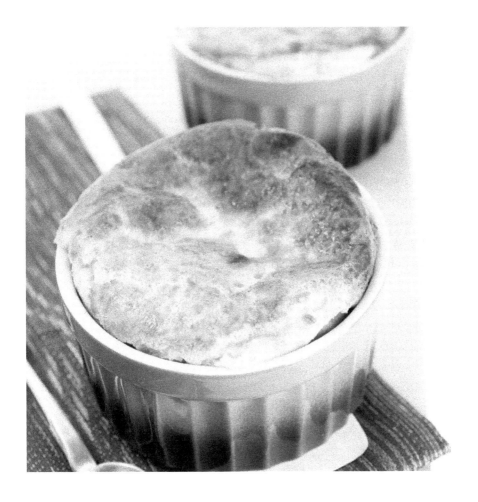

Chocolate Truffles

Preparation time: 10 minutes
Cooking time: 5 minutes
Makes: 16 truffles

Ingredients:

¼ cup full-fat coconut milk
5 ounces (142 g) sugar-free dark chocolate, finely chopped
1 tablespoon solid coconut oil, at room temperature
¼ cup unsweetened cocoa powder, for coating
Line the baking sheet with parchment paper and set aside.

Directions:

In the small saucepan, heat the coconut milk over medium heat for about 3 minutes, until hot. Stir in the chocolate and let sit in the coconut milk until beginning to melt. When most of the chocolate has softened, stir carefully with a whisk until all of the chocolate is melted and the texture is smooth and glossy. Add the coconut oil and stir gently until combined.

Transfer the mixture to the medium airtight container and refrigerate until firm and set, about 30 minutes.

Using a small cookie scoop or spoon, scoop out the truffles, about 1 inch in diameter each, and shape lightly in your hands. Move quickly, and only lightly touch the chocolate or it will begin to melt in your hands.

Roll the truffles in the cocoa powder and place on the lined baking sheet. Refrigerate for another 10 minutes to set before serving.

Store leftovers in an airtight container in the refrigerator for up to 3 days or freeze for up to 3 weeks.

Nutrition:

(1 Truffle) calories 75, fat 6.0g, protein 2.0g, carbs 3.0g, net carbs 1.0g, fiber 2.0g

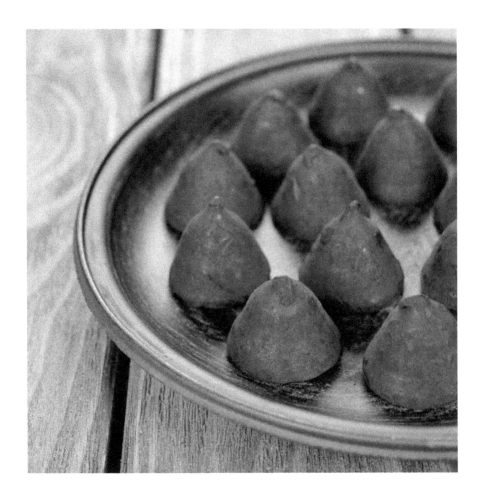

Rice Pudding

Preparation time: 10 minutes
Cooking time: 2 hours
Servings: 6

Ingredients:
tablespoon butter
7 ounces long grain rice
4 ounces water
16 ounces milk
3 ounces sugar
1 egg
1 tablespoon cream
1 teaspoon vanilla extract

Directions:
In your slow cooker, mix butter with rice, water, milk, sugar, egg, cream and vanilla, stir, cover and cook on High for 2 hours.
Stir pudding one more time, divide into bowls and serve.

Nutrition:
Calories 152, Fat 4, Fiber 4, Carbs 6, Protein 4

Drinks

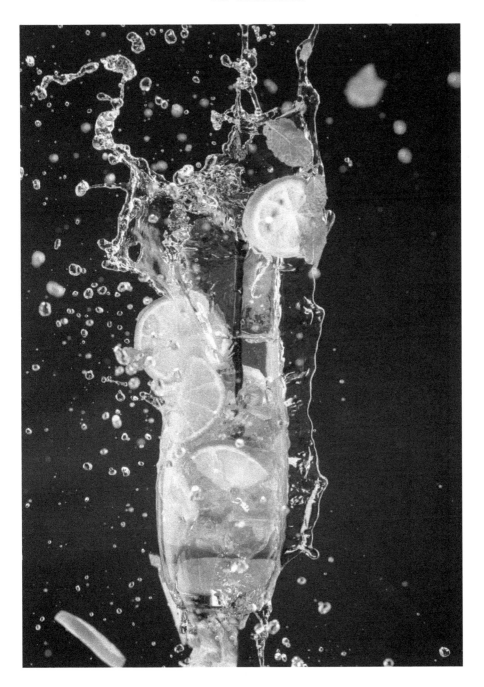

Basil Pesto

Preparation time: 5 minutes
Cooking time: 0 minutes
Makes: ¾ cup

Ingredients:

1 cup fresh basil leaves
¼ cup extra-virgin olive oil
¼ cup grated Parmesan cheese
¼ cup pine nuts
1 tablespoon chopped garlic
¼ teaspoon kosher salt
⅛ teaspoon ground black pepper

Direction:

Put all of the ingredients in a small blender or mini food processor. Pulse until fully combined but not quite smooth. Store in an airtight container in the refrigerator for up to 1 week or in the freezer for up to 3 months.

Nutrition:

calories 140, fat 14.0g, protein 2.9g, carbs 1.4g, net carbs 1.0g, fiber 0.4g

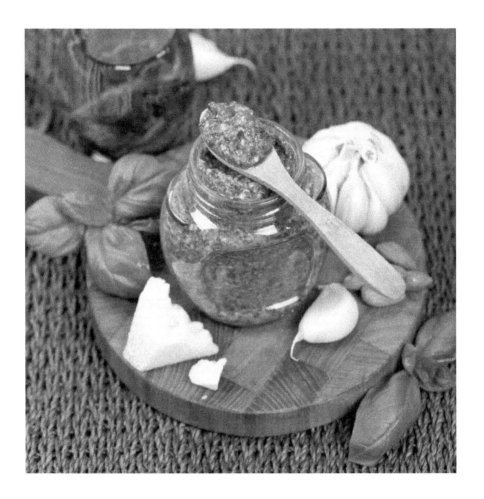

Chicken Seasoning

Preparation time: 5 minutes
Cooking time: 0 minutes
Makes: ¾ cup

Ingredients:
2 tablespoons dried parsley
2 tablespoons kosher salt
2 tablespoons onion powder
2 tablespoons smoked paprika
1 tablespoon dried rosemary leaves
1 tablespoon dried thyme leaves
tablespoon garlic powder
teaspoons ground black pepper

Directions:
Place all of the ingredients in a small bowl and mix well. Store in an airtight container for up to 6 months.

Nutrition:
calories 5, fat 0g, protein 0g, carbs 1.6g, net carbs 1.0g, fiber 0.6g

Alfredo Sauce

Preparation time: 5 minutes
Cooking time: 1 minutes
Makes: 1½ cups

Ingredients:

½ cup mascarpone cheese (4 ounces / 113 g)

¼ cup grated Parmesan cheese

¼ cup (½ stick) butter

½ cup heavy whipping cream

½ teaspoon kosher salt

¼ teaspoon ground black pepper

Directions:

Place the mascarpone, Parmesan, and butter in a medium-sized microwave-safe bowl. Microwave on high for 30 seconds, then stir.

Microwave on high for 30 seconds more. Add the cream, salt, and pepper to the bowl. Whisk together until smooth. Serve immediately.

Nutrition:

calories 240, fat 23.9g, protein 3.1g, carbs 1.2g, net carbs 1.2g, fiber 0g

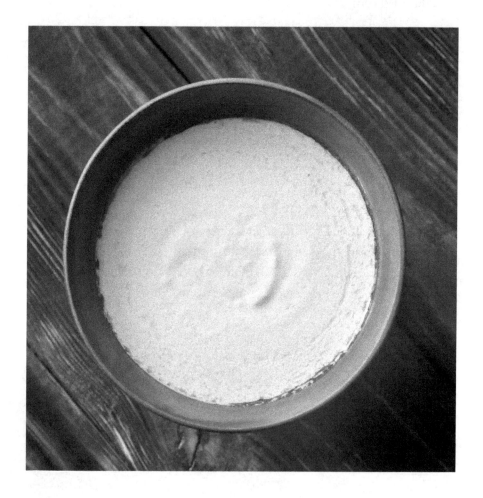

Blue Cheese Dressing

Preparation time: 5 minutes
Cooking time: 0 minutes
Makes: 1 cup

Ingredients:

⅓ cup sugar-free mayonnaise
¼ cup crumbled blue cheese
ounce (28 g) cream cheese (2 tablespoons), softened
tablespoons heavy whipping cream
1 teaspoon lemon juice

Directions:

Place all of the ingredients in a small blender and blend for 30 seconds, until creamy and nearly entirely smooth. Store in an airtight container in the refrigerator for up to 1 week.

Nutrition:

calories 101, fat 10.2g, protein 1.0g, carbs 0.5g, net carbs 0.5g, fiber 0g

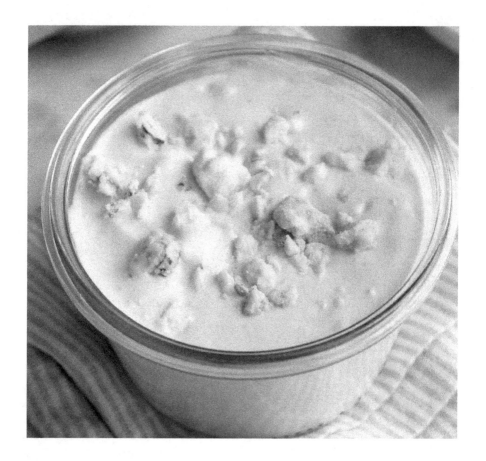

Sriracha Sauce

Preparation time: 5 minutes
Cooking time: 0 minutes
Makes: ¾ cup

Ingredients:

½ cup sugar-free mayonnaise

1½ tablespoons lime juice

1½ tablespoons Sriracha sauce

1 tablespoon granulated erythritol

Directions:

Place all of the ingredients in a small bowl and stir well until combined. Store in an airtight container in the refrigerator for up to 1 week.

Nutrition:

calories 140, fat 15.8g, protein 0g, carbs 1.0g, net carbs 1.0g, fiber 0g

Seafood Seasoning

Preparation time: 5 minutes
Cooking time: 0 minutes
Servings: ½ cup

Ingredients:
3 tablespoons dried parsley
1 tablespoon dried chives
1 tablespoon dried dill weed
tablespoon grated lemon zest
teaspoons celery salt
1 teaspoon dried marjoram leaves
1 teaspoon garlic powder
1 teaspoon ground coriander
1 teaspoon kosher salt
1 teaspoon onion powder
1 teaspoon paprika
½ teaspoon ground white pepper

Directions:
Place all of the ingredients in a small bowl and mix well. Store in an airtight container for up to 6 months.

Nutrition:
calories 2, fat 0g, protein 0g, carbs 1.5g, net carbs 1.0g, fiber 0.5g

Other Keto Recipes

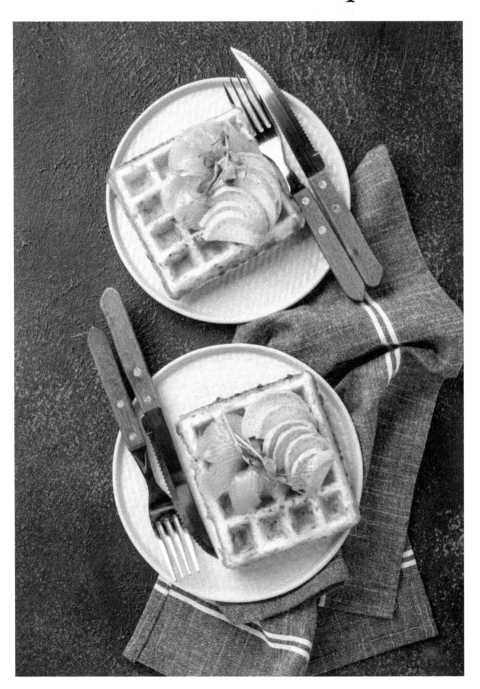

Muffin with Broccoli and Cheese

Preparation Time: 15 minutes
Cooking Time: 20 minutes
Servings: 6

Ingredients:
2 tablespoons unsalted butter
6 large organic eggs
1/2 cup heavy whipping cream
1/2 cup Parmesan cheese, grated
Salt and ground black pepper, as required
11/4 cups broccoli, chopped
2 tablespoons fresh parsley, chopped
1/2 cup Swiss cheese, grated

Directions:
Grease a 12-cup muffin tin. In a bowl or container, put in the cream, eggs, Parmesan cheese, salt, and black pepper, and beat until well combined. Divide the broccoli and parsley in the bottom of each prepared muffin cup evenly. Top with the egg mixture, followed by the Swiss cheese. Let the muffins bake for about 20 minutes, rotating the pan once halfway through. Carefully, invert the muffins onto a serving platter and serve warm.

Nutrition:
calories 241, fat 11.5g, fiber 8.5g, carbohydrates 4.1 g, protein: 11.1g

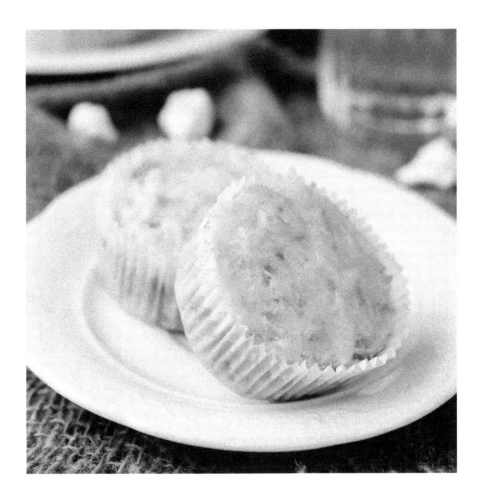

Stewed Duck Breast

Preparation time: 15 minutes
Cooking time: 25 minutes
Servings: 3

Ingrediens:

2 teaspoons canola oil
1 red bell pepper, deveined and chopped
1 shallot, chopped
½ cup celery rib, chopped
½ cup chayote, peeled and cubed
1 pound (454 g) duck breasts, boneless, skinless, and chopped into small chunks
1½ cups vegetable broth
½ stick Mexican cinnamon
1 thyme sprig
1 rosemary sprig

Directions:

Sea salt and freshly ground black pepper, to taste
Heat the canola oil in a soup pot (or clay pot) over a medium-high flame. Now, sauté the bell pepper, shallot and celery until they have softened about 5 minutes.
Add the remaining ingredients and stir to combine. Once it starts boiling, turn the heat to simmer and partially cover the pot.
Let it simmer for 17 to 20 minutes or until thoroughly cooked. Enjoy!

Nutritions:

calories: 230, fat: 9.6g, protein: 30.5g, carbs: 3.3g, net carbs: 2.3g, fiber: 1

Meat Pie

Preparation Time: 5 minutes
Cooking Time: 3-9 minutes
Servings: 2

Ingredients:
1/4 cup olive oil
1-pound grass-fed ground beef
1/2 cup celery, chopped
1/4 cup yellow onion, chopped
3 garlic cloves, minced
cup tomatoes, chopped
(12-ounce) packages riced cauliflower, cooked and well-drained
1 cup cheddar cheese, shredded
1/4 cup Parmesan cheese, shredded
1 cup heavy cream
1 teaspoon dried thyme

Directions:
Preheat your oven to 350°F.
Heat oil heat and cook the ground beef, celery, onions, and garlic for about 8–10 minutes. Immediately stir in the tomatoes. Transfer mixture into a 10x7-inch casserole dish evenly. In a food processor, add the cauliflower, cheeses, cream, thyme, and pulse until a mashed potatoes-like mixture is formed. Spread the cauliflower mixture over the meat in the casserole dish evenly. Bake for about 35–40 minutes. Cut into desired sized pieces and serve.

Nutrition:
calories 387, fat 11.5g, fiber 9.4g, carbohydrates 5.5 g, protein 18.5g

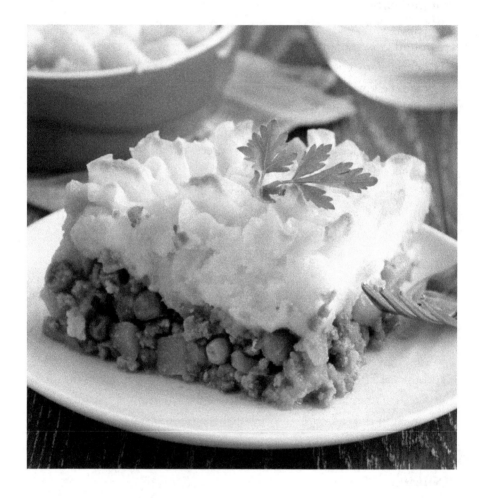

Keto Beef Casserole

Preparation time: 15 minutes
Cooking time: 4 hours
Servings: 6

Ingredients:
tablespoon olive oil
pounds (907 g) ground beef
head broccoli, cut into florets
Salt and black pepper, to taste
teaspoons mustard
2 teaspoons Worcestershire sauce
28 ounces (794 g) canned diced tomatoes
2 cups Mozzarella cheese, grated
16 ounces (454 g) tomato sauce
2 tablespoons fresh parsley, chopped
1 teaspoon dried oregano

Directions:
Apply black pepper and salt to the broccoli florets, set them into a bowl, drizzle over the olive oil, and toss well to coat completely. In a separate bowl, combine the beef with Worcestershire sauce, salt, mustard, and black pepper, and stir well. Press on the slow cooker's bottom.
Scatter in the broccoli, add the tomatoes, parsley, Mozzarella, oregano, and tomato sauce.
Cook for 4 hours on low; covered. Split the casserole among bowls and enjoy while hot.

Nutrition:
calories 435, fat 21.1g, protein 50.9g, carbs 13.5g, net carbs 5.5g, fiber 8.0g

Tuna Meatballs

Preparation Time: 15 minutes
Cooking Time: 10 minutes
Servings: 2

Ingredients:
(15-ounce) can water-packed tuna, drained
1/2 celery stalk, chopped
tablespoon fresh parsley, chopped
teaspoon fresh dill, chopped
tablespoons walnuts, chopped
2 tablespoons mayonnaise
1 organic egg, beaten
1 tablespoon butter
3 cups lettuce

Directions:
For burgers: Add all ingredients (except the butter and lettuce) in a bowl and mix until well combined.
Make two equal-sized patties from the mixture.
Melt some butter and cook the patties for about 2–3 minutes.
Carefully flip the side and cook for about 2–3 minutes.
Divide the lettuce onto serving plates.
Top each plate with one burger and serve.

Nutrition:
calories: 267, fat: 12.5g, fiber: 9.4g, carbohydrates: 3.8 g, protein: 11.5g

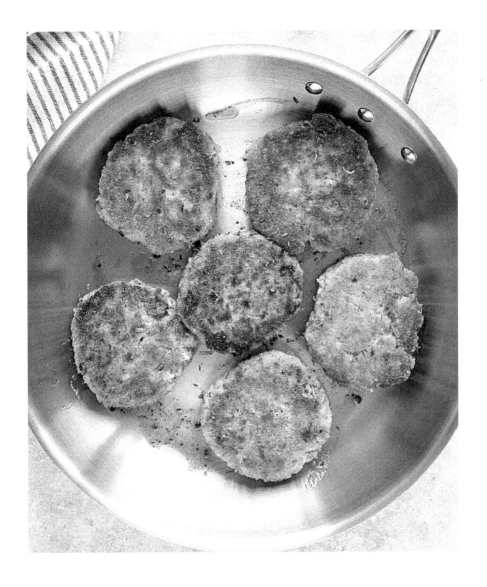

Leek and Cabbage Salad

Preparation time: 15 minutes
Cooking time: 40 minutes
Servings: 4

Ingredients:
3 tablespoons extra-virgin olive oil
1 medium-sized leek, chopped
½ pound (227 g) green cabbage, shredded
½ teaspoon caraway seeds
Sea salt, to taste
4-5 black peppercorns
1 garlic clove, minced
1 teaspoon yellow mustard
1 tablespoon balsamic vinegar
½ teaspoon Sriracha sauce

Directions:
Drizzle 2 tablespoons of the olive oil over the leek and cabbage;
sprinkle with caraway seeds, salt, black peppercorns.
Roast in the preheated oven at 420°F (216°C) for 37 to 40 minutes.
Place the roasted mixture in a salad bowl.
Toss with the remaining tablespoon of olive oil garlic, mustard,
vinegar, and Sriracha sauce. Serve immediately and enjoy!

Nutrition:
calories 116, fat 10.1g, protein 1.0g, carbs 6.5g, net carbs 4.7g,
fiber 1.8g

Garlicky Coconut Milk and Tomato Soup

Preparation time: 15 minutes
Cooking time: 30 minutes
Servings: 6

Ingredients:
6 cups vegetable broth
½ cup full-fat unsweetened coconut milk
1½ cups canned diced tomatoes
1 yellow onion, chopped
3 cloves garlic, chopped
1 teaspoon Italian seasoning
1 bay leaf

Directions:
Pinch of salt and pepper, to taste
Fresh basil, for serving
Add all the ingredients minus the coconut milk and fresh basil to a stockpot over medium heat and bring to a boil. Reduce to a simmer and cook for 30 minutes.
Remove the bay leaf, and then use an immersion blender to blend the soup until smooth. Stir in the coconut milk.
Garnish with fresh basil and serve.

Nutrition:
calories 105, fat 6.9g, protein 6.1g, carbs 5.8g, net carbs 4.8g, fiber 1.0g

Tex-Mex Queso Dip

Preparation Time: 5 minutes
Cooking Time: 10 minutes
Servings: 6

Ingredients:
1/2 cup of coconut milk
1/2 jalapeño pepper, seeded and diced
teaspoon minced garlic
1/2 teaspoon onion powder
ounces goat cheese
6 ounces sharp Cheddar cheese, shredded
1/4 teaspoon cayenne pepper

Directions:
Preheat a pot then add the coconut milk, jalapeño, garlic, and onion powder.
Simmer then whisk in the goat cheese until smooth.
Add the Cheddar cheese and cayenne and whisk until the dip is thick, 30 seconds to 1 minute.

Nutrition:
calories 149, fat 12.1g, fiber 3.1g, carbohydrates 5.1 g, protein 4.2g

Southern Pecan

Preparation time: 5 minutes
Cooking time: 15 minutes
Makes: 18 clusters

Ingredients:
4 tablespoons (½ stick) unsalted butter, at room temperature
¼ cup granulated erythritol–monk fruit blend
1½ cups pecan halves
½ teaspoon salt
2 tablespoons heavy whipping cream

Directions:
Line the baking sheet with parchment paper and set aside.
In the skillet, melt the butter over medium-high heat. Using the silicone spatula, stir in the erythritol–monk fruit blend and combine well, making sure to dissolve the sugar in the butter. Stir in the pecan halves and salt.
Once the pecans are completely covered in the glaze, add the heavy cream and quickly stir. When the heavy cream bubbles and evaporates, remove from the heat immediately. Quickly spoon the clusters of 4 to 5 pecan halves each onto the prepared baking sheet and allow to fully cool and set, 15 to 20 minutes, before enjoying.
Store leftovers in an airtight container on the counter or in the refrigerator for up 5 days.

Nutrition:
(1 Cluster) calories 86, fat 9.0g, protein 1.0g, carbs 1.0g, net carbs 0g, fiber 1.0g

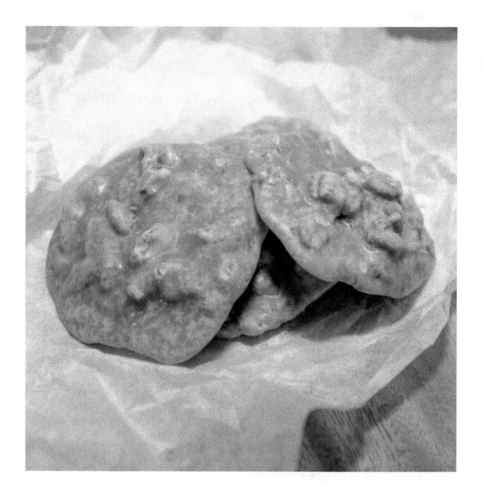

Coconut Cheesecake

Preparation Time: 15 minutes
Cooking Time: 25 minutes
Servings: 12

Ingredients:
Crust:
 egg whites
1/4 cup erythritol
cups desiccated coconut
1 tsp. coconut oil
1/4 cup melted butter

Filling:
3 tbsp. lemon juice
6 ounces raspberries
2 cups erythritol
1 cup whipped cream
Zest of 1 lemon
24 ounces cream cheese

Directions:
Line the pan with parchment paper. Preheat oven to 350°F and mix all
crust ingredients. Pour the crust into the pan. Bake for about 25
minutes; let cool.
Whisk the cream cheese in a container. Add the lemon juice, zest, and
erythritol. Fold in whipped cream mixture. Fold in the raspberries
gently. Spoon the filling into the crust. Place in the fridge for 4 hours.

Nutrition:
calories 214, fat 11.4g, fiber 8.4g, carbohydrates 5.4g, protein: 9.1g

CPSIA information can be obtained
at www.ICGtesting.com
Printed in the USA
BVHW091511100621
609271BV00004B/1154